AMPUTATIONS AND PROSTHETICS
A Case Study Approach

AMPUTATIONS AND PROSTHETICS
A Case Study Approach

Bella J. May, EdD, PT, FAPTA
Professor
Department of Physical Therapy
Medical College of Georgia
and
President
BJM Enterprises, PC
Augusta, Georgia

 F. A. DAVIS COMPANY • Philadelphia

F. A. Davis Company
1915 Arch Street
Philadelphia, PA 19103

Printed in the United States of America

Last digit indicates print number: 10 9 8 7 6 5 4

Publisher: Jean-François Vilain
Developmental Editor: Ralph Zickgraf
Production Editor: Jessica Howie Martin
Cover Designer: Steven Ross Morrone

As new scientific information becomes available through basic and clinical research, recommended treatments and drug therapies undergo changes. The author and publisher have done everything possible to make this book accurate, up to date, and in accord with accepted standards at the time of publication. The author, editors, and publisher are not responsible for errors or omissions or for consequences from application of the book, and make no warranty, expressed or implied, in regard to the contents of the book. Any practice described in this book should be applied by the reader in accordance with professional standards of care used in regard to the unique circumstances that may apply in each situation. The reader is advised always to check product information (package inserts) for changes and new information regarding dose and contraindications before administering any drug. Caution is especially urged when using new or infrequently ordered drugs.

Library of Congress Cataloging-in-Publication Data

May, Bella J.
    Amputations and prosthetics : a case study approach / by Bella J. May.
      p.   cm.
    Includes bibliographical references and index.
    ISBN 0-8036-0043-7 (pbk.)
    1. Amputation—Physical therapy—Case studies.   2. Amputees—Rehabilitation—Case studies.   3. Artificial limbs—Case studies.
4. Prosthesis—Case studies.   5. Extremities (Anatomy)—Amputation—Case studies. I. Title.
    [DNLM: 1. Amputation—rehabilitation. 2. Prosthesis. 3. Physical Therapy—methods. 4. Amputees—psychology. WE 170 M466a 1996]
    RD553.M425   1996
    617.5'803—dc20
    DNLM/DLC
    for Library of Congress   96-15601

Preface

The number of individuals surviving amputation for vascular disease, malignant tumors, and serious trauma is increasing. People with amputations want to return to an active lifestyle. In past years, clients who had an amputation were often referred to specialized clinics for postsurgical care and prosthetic rehabilitation. Today they receive treatment in local hospitals, outpatient centers, rehabilitation facilities, extended care facilities, and the home. Many are elderly persons who present with multiple physical problems but who are not content to remain in a wheelchair after amputation. Most physical therapists (PTs) and physical therapist assistants (PTAs) provide services to individuals who have sustained one or more amputations as a regular part of their practice.

The field of prosthetics has undergone major growth in the past several decades. Bioengineering research has led to the development of prosthetic components that duplicate many of the complex functions of both lower and upper extremities. There are prosthetic feet that provide varying degrees of dynamic response and mechanical and hydraulic knee mechanisms, some computer-driven, that respond to the mobility demands of both active and sedentary clients. PTs and PTAs must understand the functions and capabilities of these devices to properly help the client learn to walk again.

Educational programs for PTs or PTAs prepare the practitioner to work effectively with people of all ages who have undergone amputations. This book is the result of teaching activities with such students for the past 25 years.

The book is designed to provide the student with the opportunity to learn the basic concepts necessary to plan and implement treatment programs following amputation. It incorporates the philosophy that active learning is more effective than passive learning and that working through simulated case studies helps the student integrate rather than memorize concepts. The book is also designed to be an effective tool for the faculty, regardless of experience in the area of amputations and prosthetics.

The first chapter provides a brief historical perspective on both physical therapy and the field of prosthetics. The second chapter introduces concepts related to the client with vascular disease and the third focuses on diabetic foot problems. These chapters have been included since the majority of clients lose a limb because of vascular insufficiency, and prevention of amputation and care of the remaining extremity are an integral part of physical therapy. The fourth chapter provides an overview of surgical processes, focusing on concepts necessary for effective postsurgical care, which is the topic of Chapter Five. The psychosocial issues related to the loss of a limb are explored in Chapter Six. Chapter Seven attempts to take the complex world of prosthetic components and make it manageable. There is no intent to cover all possible prosthetic components. Rather, the chapter attempts to guide the reader through the labyrinth and provide a basis for later integration of newer items as they become available. Chapter Eight presents a motor control approach to prosthetic checkout and training and Chapter Nine reviews long term management. Occasionally a PT or PTA may be involved in the care of an individual following upper extremity amputation or may work with a child who has a congenital or acquired amputation. Chapters Ten and Eleven are there as references for these subjects when needed.

The book is designed to be used in educational programs that include amputations and prosthetics as part of other courses as well as programs that have a separate course. As a text for both PTs and PTAs, it may contain concepts and activities beyond the scope of practice of the PTA. However, understanding each other's scope of practice may help both PTs and PTAs later in the work setting. The book is also a reference for practitioners who want to review the latest evaluation and treatment concepts as well as increase their knowledge of new components. Working with individuals with amputations is challenging and exciting; I hope students and practitioners enjoy it as much as I have.

Bella J. May

Acknowledgments

Many people have contributed to the creation and development of this book. Particular thanks go to the reviewers who labored over rough drafts, making valuable suggestions for improvements. The following individuals reviewed all or part of the manuscript:

P. W. Dent, MS, PT
Assistant Professor and Director, Physical Therapist Assistant Program
Massachusetts Bay Community College
Wellesley Hills, Massachusetts

Joan E. Edelstein, MA, PT, FISPO
Associate Professor of Clinical Physical Therapy and Director, Program in Physical Therapy
Columbia University
New York, New York

G. William Limehouse, CP
Regional Manager
J. E. Hanger Company
Augusta, Georgia

Eleanor J. Repetto, PT, MBA
Director, Physical Therapist Assistant Program
Newbury College
Brookline, Massachusetts

Neil D. Schuster, MS, PT
Division Director Physical Therapy
Maine Medical Center
Portland, Maine

Thanks also go to Gloria T. Sanders, BS, MS, PT, Owner, Onslow Rehabilitation Center, Hubert, North Carolina, for authorization to use her illustrations from the book *Lower Limb Amputations: A Guide to Rehabilitation.*

Particular thanks go to the J. E. Hanger Company of Augusta, Georgia. William Limehouse, CP, Regional Manager, and Robert Edwards, CP, Augusta Officer Manager, as well as the staff of the facility, have long assisted me with teaching materials and suggestions as well as components and people for "one more picture."

The Physical Therapy Class of 1996 and my fellow faculty member, Thomas L. Stec, MHE, PT, from the Medical College of Georgia served as testers of the final product. They provided valuable feedback, as have all students over the past 25 years. Cecelia King, Administrative Coordinator in the Department of Physical Therapy of the Medical College of Georgia, assisted with printing, scanning photographs, making phone calls, and generally supporting a demanding author.

I am grateful to the many clients who willingly let their pictures be taken and used in this book and in teaching slides and videotapes. I am also grateful to the many clients who have taught me so much in 43 years of practice.

Bella J. May

Contributors

Jeffrey S. Dowling, MHE, PT
Assistant Director
Department of Physical Therapy
Medical College of Georgia Hospitals and Clinics
Augusta, Georgia

Joan E. Edelstein, MA, PT, FISPO
Associate Professor of Clinical Physical Therapy and
Director, Program in Physical Therapy
Columbia University
New York, New York

Contents

chapter one

Amputations and Prosthetics: Then and Now

OBJECTIVES

At the end of this chapter, all students are expected to:

1 Discuss the key milestones in the history of amputations and prosthetics.
2 Discuss elements and events that triggered improvements in rehabilitation of individuals with amputations.
3 Discuss the composition of the prosthetic clinic team.
4 Discuss the role and function of members of the amputee clinic team.

Imagine that it is 1925 and you are studying physical therapy at Harvard University. You graduated from Radcliffe College with a degree in physical education last June and decided to enroll in a certificate course in physical therapeutics. You became interested in that field when your brother Brian lost his right leg below the knee in 1918 during World War I. You went to the hospital several times and watched Brian learning to use a wooden leg under the guidance of a reconstruction aide. Reconstruction aides were women who had completed a special 6 month course in physical therapeutics after obtaining a college degree, usually in physical education. The prosthesis, as the leg is now called, was carved from a block of willow wood by a prosthetist who himself had had an amputation. The residual limb (then called a stump) fit into a cylinder held on by a long leather corset with metal uprights that fit around the thigh. The prosthesis had a wooden foot with rubber bumpers to simulate dorsiflexion and plantar flexion (Fig. 1.1). It weighed about 9 pounds.

Now, in 1925, you are learning to be a physical therapist. You learn to teach people with amputations to toughen their residual limbs by tapping on the skin with a soda bottle wrapped in a towel or with the fingertips. You also learn about wooden legs. In 1925, there are few people with amputations. Most are

1

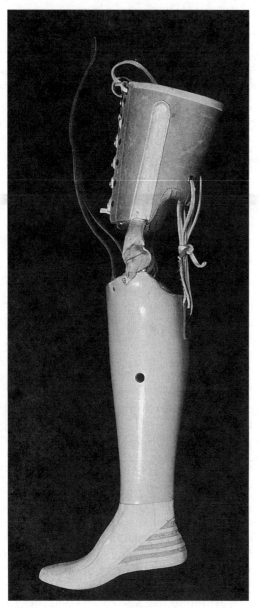

FIGURE 1.1
Conventional transtibial prosthesis similar in style to the prostheses used until the 1950s. (With permission from Sanders, GT: Lower Limb Amputations: A Guide to Rehabilitation. FA Davis, Philadelphia, 1986.)

young because amputations are usually performed because of some kind of trauma, such as a war wound or an accident.

Move now to the present. You are a physical therapist or physical therapist assistant student learning about amputations and prosthetics. You may have a relative or an acquaintance who has lost a leg. It is likely that this person had an amputation because of peripheral vascular disease and ischemia of the lower leg. He or she may have diabetes and will probably be over age 60. The prosthesis is made of plastic and may have been fabricated by a computer from an electronic image of the residual limb. The prosthesis is held on by a light elastic sleeve that rolls over the thigh or the high plastic wings of the prosthesis. The

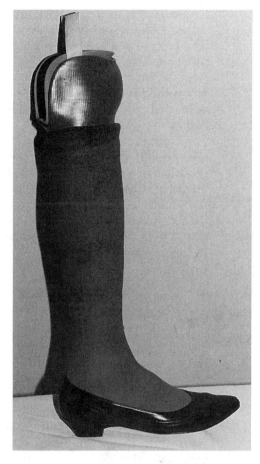

FIGURE 1.2
Modern patellar tendon bearing, suprapatellar, supracondylar endoskeleton transtibial prosthesis.

shank is a lightweight aluminum pipe covered with a soft covering shaped to resemble the other leg. The foot is designed to simulate the push off of the normal foot (Fig. 1.2). The entire leg weighs less than 3 pounds.

CASE STUDY ACTIVITIES

1   Review the historical developments presented in this chapter. In study groups, discuss the changes that have occurred, and the impetus for those changes, and become familiar with some of the terminology. Consider the future. What do you think are the important concepts to understand to be effective as a physical therapist or physical therapist assistant?

2   If various prostheses are available, examine and handle them to gain a better understanding of the effect of technological advances.

History

The earliest amputations usually resulted in death from shock caused by blood loss or septicemia. Those who survived the operation itself often died in the early postoperative period of infection and gangrene. The emphasis was on surgical speed rather than shaping the residual limb. When antisepsis and anesthesia came into use in the mid 19th century, specific surgical techniques, tissue conservation, and postoperative management became the focus of amputation surgery. From the first amputation recorded in history, performed by Hegesistratus in 484 BC, prosthetic replacements have been designed to improve function. Hegesistratus, who escaped from the stocks by cutting off one of his feet, built himself a wooden foot to compensate. There are records of 15th century knights who built and used iron artificial hands to hold their swords.[1]

Over the years, attempts to improve function have resulted in technical advances in artificial limbs and attempts to save lives have brought about surgical improvements. Changes in technology and materials have led to improvements in surgery and prosthetics. Government legislation has also contributed, particularly after wars, when government agencies provided funds for prosthetic research. A brief chronological look at the major historical developments in the field of amputation and prosthetics will help to place current concepts in perspective.

THE EARLY YEARS

Surgery

In the early years, there were more changes in surgical techniques than in prosthetics. Operative and postoperative bleeding was a major problem. In 1517, Hans von Gersdorff of Strassburg described the use of a compression tourniquet and cauterization to control bleeding.[2] He also recommended covering an amputated limb with muscle from a cow's or pig's bladder and dressing the wound with warm (not boiling) oil. Ambroise Paré[3] (1510–1590), a French army surgeon, reintroduced the use of ligatures, originally described by Hippocrates. This technique was more successful than crushing the amputation limb, dipping it in boiling oil, or other means of cautery that had been used during the Dark Ages to stop bleeding. Paré was the first to describe phantom sensation. Wilhelm Fabry[2] of Germany first recommended amputation above a gangrenous part. He devised a tourniquet (a ligature tightened by a stick) to stop circulation before surgery. In 1803, Dominique Jean Larrey,[2] Napoleon's surgeon, tried refrigeration to dull the pain of amputation surgery. He was one of the first to amputate at the hip joint. He was said to have performed as many as 200 amputations in 24 hours and is recognized as the inventor of "flying ambulances," with which he gathered wounded men during battle rather than compelling them to wait until the end of the conflict. In 1815, Jacques Lisfranc[3] of France devised a disarticulation amputation of the foot at the tarsometatarsal joint that became known as Lisfranc's amputation.

James Syme[3] of Edinburgh performed the first successful amputation at the ankle joint in 1842; the procedure carries his name. He also advocated thigh amputations through the cortical bone of the condyles or the trochanters. That same year, Crawford Long,[3] who practiced in Athens, Georgia, was the first physician to use ether for general anesthesia. Pierre Jean Marie Flourens,[1] a French physiologist, discovered the anesthetic properties of chloroform in 1847. The increasing availability of ether and chloroform led to improved surgical procedures and more functional residual limbs. In 1867, Joseph Lister[2] published a book on his principles of antiseptic surgery, which markedly reduced mortality during and after surgery. Lister also experimented with using catgut as a ligature (1880) rather than silk or hemp, which were not absorbed by bodily tissues and often caused inflammations and hemorrhage. In the early 1900s, surgeons attempted to build bone bridges at the ends of transtibial (below knee) amputations to allow greater end bearing. These techniques were precursors of the development of myodesis and myoplasty techniques discussed later in this chapter and in Chapter 4.

In 1848, Vanghetti, an Italian surgeon, attempted to develop a technique to power an upper limb prosthesis directly using muscles attached to the prosthesis.[1] The technique was further refined in Germany and Argentina as surgeons developed skin lined muscle tunnels, an early cineplasty, to power upper limb prostheses.[1]

Prosthetics

Early prosthetic developments are not as well documented. It is likely that prostheses were made by local artisans or individuals who were themselves in need

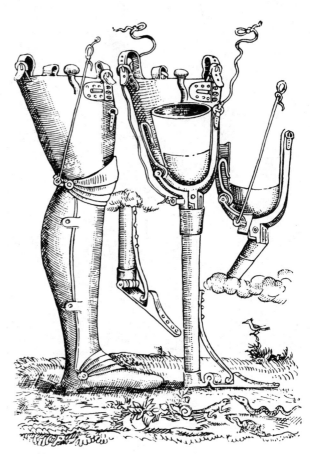

FIGURE 1.3
An above knee artificial leg invented by Ambroise Paré (middle sixteenth century). (From Paré, A: Oeuvres Complètes, Paris, 1840. From the copy in the National Library of Medicine.)

of such limbs. An artificial leg invented by Paré in 1561 for individuals whose legs had been amputated above the knee was constructed of iron and was the first artificial leg known to employ articulated joints (Fig. 1.3). In 1696, Pieter Andriannszoon Verfuyn (Verduin),[2,3] a Dutch surgeon, introduced the first known transtibial prosthesis with an unlocked knee joint. In concept, it resembled the thigh/corset prosthesis used in more recent times. A thigh cuff bore part of the weight and was connected by external hinges to a leg piece whose socket was made of copper and lined with leather. The leg piece terminated in a wooden foot. In 1843, James Potts[3] of London introduced a transfemoral (above knee) prosthesis with a wooden shank and socket, a steel knee joint, and an articulated foot with leather thongs connecting the knee to the ankle. This enabled dorsiflexion (toe lift) whenever the wearer flexed the knee. The device was known as the "Anglesey (Anglesea) leg" because it was used by the Marquis of Anglesey after the loss of his leg in the Battle of Watterloo (Fig. 1.4).

During the American Civil War, from 1861 to 1865, interest in artificial limbs and amputation surgery increased because of the number of individuals who survived amputations (30,000 in the Union army alone) and the commitment of federal and state governments to pay for artificial limbs for veterans. J. E. Hanger,[3] who lost a leg during the Civil War, replaced the cords of his prosthesis with rubber bumpers at the ankle to control plantar flexion and dor-

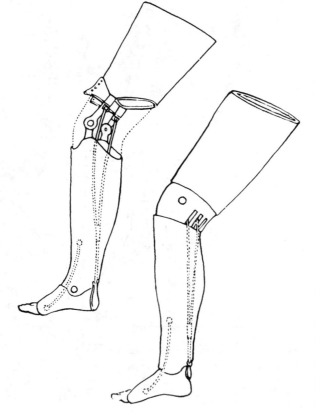

FIGURE 1.4

The Anglesey (Anglesea) leg (1816) with articulated knee, ankle, and foot. (*Left*) Below knee. (*Right*) Above knee. (From Bigg, HH: Orthopraxy: The Mechanical Treatment of Deformities, Debilities and Deficiencies of the Human Frame, ed 3. J & A Churchill, London, 1877.)

siflexion. The J. E. Hanger Company opened in Richmond, Virginia in 1861, and in 1862, the first law providing free prostheses to people who had lost limbs in warfare was enacted by the United States Congress.[3]

In 1863 the suction socket (Fig. 1.5), which employed the concept of using pressure to suspend an artificial limb, was patented by an American, Dubois D. Parmelee,[4] who also invented a polycentric knee unit and a multiarticulated foot. In 1870, Congress passed a law that not only supplied artificial limbs to all honorably discharged persons from the military or naval service who had lost a limb while in the United States service, but also entitled them to receive a new one every 5 years.

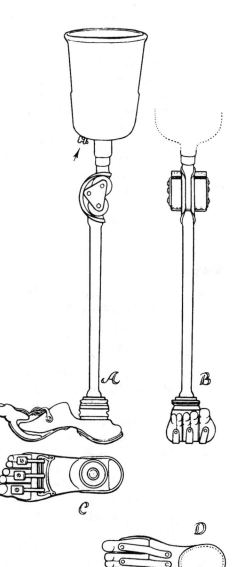

FIGURE 1.5
The D. D. Parmelee prosthesis with suction socket, patented in 1863. (With permission from Historical development of artificial limbs. In Orthopaedic Appliances Atlas, Vol 2, Artificial Limbs. JW Edwards, Ann Arbor, 1960, p. 11.)

THE WORLD WARS

Only 4403 American soldiers lost limbs during World War I (1914 to 1918), compared with 42,000 British soldiers. The total number of amputations in all of the armies of Europe was approximately 100,000. The war was, however, an impetus for improvements in artificial limb development.[5] Collaboration between prosthetists and surgeons in the care of veterans with amputations led to the formation of the Artificial Limb Manufacturers Association in 1917. Little progress was made in the field of prosthetics and amputation surgery in the period between the two wars, but World War II again spurred developments. The American Orthotics and Prosthetics Association (AOPA) was established in 1949 and developed educational criteria and examinations to certify prosthetists and orthotists.[3]

In 1945, in response to the demands of veterans for more functional prostheses, the National Academy of Sciences (NAS) initiated a study to develop design criteria for artificial limbs that would improve function.[1] The Committee on Artificial Limbs (CAL) contracted with universities, industrial laboratories, health providers, and others to spearhead major changes in all facets of prosthetics and orthotics. From 1947 to 1976, under NAS sponsorship and Veterans Administration (VA) support, the CAL, the Committee on Prosthetic Research and Development (CPRD), and the Committee on Prosthetic-Orthotic Education (CPOE) influenced the development of modern prosthetics and orthotics.[1] Plastic replaced wood as the material of choice, socket designs followed physiological principles of function, lighter weight components were developed, and more cosmetic alternatives were fabricated. Most of the prosthetic principles outlined in this book had their inception in the work of these committees.[1]

Surgery

Surgically, myoplasty (the suturing of the ends of severed muscles over the end of the bone) was first advocated in 1949,[1] but did not gain popularity until the 1950s, when it was adopted by Dederich[6] and popularized by Burgess et al.[7] Myodesis (the suturing of severed muscles to distal bone) was advocated by Weiss[8] in the 1960s. Both myodesis and myoplasty are designed to provide muscle fixation for improved function and shape of the residual limb. In 1958 Michel Berlemont, in France, demonstrated immediate postsurgical fitting of prostheses.[3] The technique, which involves placing the residual limb in a rigid postsurgical dressing fabricated according to prosthetic principles, was also advocated by Weiss[8] and brought to the United States by Sarmiento et al.[9] and Burgess et al.[7]

In the 1960s and 1970s various factors combined to lead surgeons to reconsider the transfemoral level as the level of choice for amputation of severely ischemic limbs. Immediate postoperative fitting reduced postoperative edema, allowing healing at transtibial levels even in individuals with severe ischemia. Improved circulatory evaluation techniques provided accurate information on the presence of collateral circulation. The use of the long posterior flap with its increased blood supply also added to the healing capabilities of transtibial amputations.[10] These factors all contributed to a reversal in the number of transtibial and transfemoral amputations performed for severe limb ischemia and concomitantly increased the number of individuals who became successful prosthetic ambulators.

Prosthetics

During the same period, many changes occurred in prosthetic development. In 1954 the Canadian hip disarticulation prosthesis, designed at Sunnybrook Hospital, Toronto and introduced by Colin McLaurin, allowed an individual with a hip disarticulation or hemipelvectomy to stand and walk with moving mechanical knee and hip joints.[3] The Canadian Syme prosthesis, also designed at Sunnybrook Hospital and introduced in 1955, combined the use of plastic laminates and a solid rubber foot.[3] In 1956 the solid ankle cushion heel (SACH) foot was introduced by the Biomechanics Laboratory at the University of California and became the most popular prosthetic foot.[3] In 1959 the patellar tendon bearing (PTB) prosthesis was first introduced at the University of California at Berkeley. In the same year, the Orthopedic Appliance and Limb Manufacturers Association changed its name to the American Orthotics and Prosthetics Association (AOPA).[2] In the 1960s hydraulic knee mechanisms became more prevalent. In 1971 endoskeletal prostheses with an adjustable tubular structure encased by a foam plastic material and covered by elastic hose were introduced by Otto Bock Orthopaedic Industry.[5]

The American Board for Certification of the Prosthetic and Orthopedic Appliance Industry, Inc. became the American Board for Certification in Orthotics and Prosthetics, Inc. The first undergraduate curriculum leading to a Bachelor of Science in Prosthetics and Orthotics was inaugurated at New York University in 1963. Throughout the postwar period, the rehabilitation of individuals with amputations involved the expertise of prosthetists, engineers, researchers, physicians, and therapists. Workshops were held by major prosthetic rehabilitation centers to share the increasing body of knowledge. Experience in and knowledge of prosthetic and orthotic rehabilitation became part of the residency requirements for orthopedic surgeons.

In 1970 the International Society for Prosthetics and Orthotics was founded to improve communication between researchers and clinicians throughout the world. To make international communications clearer and easier, a standard nomenclature was adopted to refer to level of amputation and related prostheses. The term **trans** is used when an amputation goes across the axis of a long bone such as the tibia (transtibial) or the humerus (transhumeral). When there are two bones together, such as the tibia and fibula, the primary bone is identified. Amputations between long bones or through a joint are referred to as disarticulations and identified by the major body part, for example, knee disarticulation. The term **partial** is used to refer to a part of the foot or hand distal to the ankle or wrist that may be amputated.[11] Table 1.1 shows the relationship between the old and new terminologies. The new terminology is used throughout this book.

MODERN TIMES

Surgery

Most amputations today are performed because of vascular disease, with more than 50 percent performed on individuals with peripheral vascular disease sec-

T A B L E 1 . 1 **AMPUTATION LEVEL NOMENCLATURE**

Old Terminology	Current Terminology
Partial hand	Partial hand
Wrist disarticulation	Wrist disarticulation
Below elbow	Transradial
Elbow disarticulation	Elbow disarticulation
Above elbow	Transhumeral
Shoulder disarticulation	Shoulder disarticulation
Forequarter	Forequarter
Partial foot	Partial foot
Syme's	Ankle disarticulation
Below knee	Transtibial
Knee disarticulation	Knee disarticulation
Above knee	Transfemoral
Hip disarticulation	Hip disarticulation
Hemipelvectomy	Transpelvic

ondary to diabetes.[12] The National Commission on Diabetes estimates that 5 to 15 percent of all persons with diabetes will require an amputation.[12] Although no recent national data on percentage of amputations by age and cause are available, by far the most prevalent cause of lower extremity amputation is vascular disease, and most amputations are performed on individuals past age 60. Trauma is the next most frequent reason for amputation, with cancer, congenital deformities, and miscellaneous causes as other reasons. In 1959 and 1960, the "thalidomide tragedy" resulted in many children born with multiple limb anomalies; this led to government-supported research, particularly in Germany, Canada, and the United States, for prostheses and aids for children with multiple amputations. Today, the major causes of juvenile amputations are trauma, congenital abnormalities, osteomyelitis, and cancer.

Limb salvage procedures, replantation, and revascularization characterize modern surgical concepts. Replantation of fingers and thumbs has been quite successful, but efforts to replant entire upper limbs have not done as well.[13] Improved techniques of fracture fixation, vessel repair, and muscle and skin flaps have enhanced limb salvage procedures. Algorithms have been developed to guide the surgeon in cases of severe multiple trauma to upper or lower limbs. Infection control has improved, and chemotherapy and tumor ablation with reconstruction have reduced the need for amputation for metastatic disease.

Prosthetics

Modern times are characterized by the emergence of prosthetics as a science as well as an art. Research into human movement, new materials, and new technology has led to the creation of light and functional components. The client is also making greater demands on the prosthesis, seeking limbs that will enable participation in all aspects of life, including sports and leisure activities. Flexible intimate fit sockets suspended by suction have been developed for trans-femoral and transtibial amputations. A variety of prosthetic feet have been designed to respond dynamically to the pressure of walking and running. Research has highlighted the importance of swing phase as well as the stance phase in normal walking, leading to the development of hydraulic and mechanical swing phase control knee joints for transfemoral amputations. Chapter 7 describes modern components for lower extremity prostheses.

The upper extremity has always posed a major challenge for prosthetists. The great complexity of hand function is difficult to duplicate mechanically. The loss of sensation limits the function of the hand or hook, and researchers have yet to develop replacement for sensory function. Research in this area is continuing. Developments in external power are probably the highlight of modern upper extremity prostheses. Myoelectric controls are now used fairly routinely for transhumeral and transradial amputations. Upper extremity prosthetics are reviewed in Chapter 10.

The Team Approach

In early times, a surgeon performed an amputation, someone made a prosthesis, and the client learned to use the appliance as best he or she could. During and after World War I, reconstruction aides taught veterans to use their prostheses, a practice that was carried into the civilian population as physical therapists became more prevalent. There is no formal documentation of the development of the prosthetic rehabilitation team. As surgeons and prosthetists started to share ideas regarding prosthetic developments and as the field of rehabilitation grew, the care of individuals following amputations became a part of the rehabilitation process in areas where rehabilitation centers existed. In smaller communities, the surgeon sent the client to a prosthetist, who made the limb. The client might or might not be referred to a physical or occupational therapist for training. As prosthetic rehabilitation became more complex, teams of experts from the fields of medicine, physical therapy, occupational therapy, prosthetics and orthotics, and social services gathered together in teams to evaluate client needs and make decisions.

Most amputations today are performed by vascular or general surgeons who may or may not have received special training in prosthetic rehabilitation. Orthopedic surgeons usually perform amputations necessitated by trauma, malignancy, or other nonvascular causes, and complete a course in prosthetics as part of their residency training. Referral to a prosthetic clinic or to physical therapy may be delayed for many weeks if the surgeon waits until the residual limb heals completely. Such delays, particularly among elderly clients, may lead to joint contractures, muscular weakness secondary to disuse, and limited mobility. Delay in starting a rehabilitation program may limit the level of rehabilitation eventually achieved. Ideally, the physical therapist should be involved before surgery, or at least immediately after, to start the process of client education, proper positioning, and residual limb care. Unfortunately, many amputations are performed in hospitals without the services of an amputee clinic or a well trained team that can develop and supervise the program. The physical therapist may be the only person with competence in prosthetic rehabilitation. Close contact with the vascular surgeons in the facility may serve to increase the likelihood of early referrals and improve quality care for the client.

TEAM MEMBERS

The clinic team plans and implements comprehensive rehabilitation programs designed to meet the physical, psychological, and economic needs of the client. Most clinic teams are located in rehabilitation facilities, university health centers, or Department of Veterans' Affairs medical centers. The team generally includes a physician, physical therapist, occupational therapist, prosthetist, social worker, and vocational counselor. Other health professionals who contribute to the team are a nurse, dietitian, psychologist, and possibly, an administrative coordinator. Table 1.2 outlines the major functions of team members. The frequency with which a clinic team meets is dictated by the caseload; clients are seen regularly and decisions are made using input from all team members. A screening session held by the physical and occupational therapists before the actual clinic meeting allows careful evaluation of each person and improves the effectiveness of the clinic.[14] In centers without a clinic, close communication among the client, surgeon, and physical therapists, with the later addition of the prosthetist, is important to ensure an optimum outcome.

SUMMARY

Major advances have been made in the field of prosthetic rehabilitation, stimulated partly by wars that increased the number of individuals who lost limbs. Dissatisfaction with heavy, uncomfortable artificial limbs, particularly after World War II, gave impetus to research in surgery and prosthetics. Today, the number of older individuals who seek a functional and productive life after amputation and the desire of all handicapped individuals for full participation in work, sports, and leisure activities continue to stimulate advances in prosthetics and rehabilitation.

T A B L E   1 . 2   **CLINIC TEAM MEMBERS AND FUNCTIONS**

Physician	Clinic chief; coordinates team decision making; supervises client's general medical condition; prescribes appliances.
Physical therapist	Evaluates and treats clients through preprosthetic and prosthetic phases; makes recommendations for prosthetic components and whether or not to fit the client. May be clinic coordinator.
Prosthetist	Fabricates and modifies prosthesis; recommends prosthetic components; shares data on new prosthetic developments.
Occupational therapist	Assesses and treats individuals with upper extremity amputations; makes recommendations for components.
Social worker	Financial counselor and coordinator; provides liaison with third party payers and community agencies; helps family cope with social and financial problems.
Dietician	Consultant for clients with diabetes or those needing diet guidance.
Vocational counselor	Assesses client's employment potential; coordinates and may fund education, training, and placement.

Source: May, BJ: Assessment and treatment of individuals following lower extremity amputation. In O'Sullivan, SB, and Schmitz, TJ (eds.): Physical Rehabilitation: Assessment and Treatment, ed 3. FA Davis, Philadelphia, 1994, with permission.

GLOSSARY

Ablation	Removal of a body part.
Amputation	Surgical removal of a limb or body part. In this text, the term is used to refer to the removal or absence of a limb.
Cauterization	Destruction of tissue by burning or freezing. Burning was once used to close wounds.
Cineplasty	A surgical technique that builds a tunnel through a muscle of the residual limb to power an artificial limb, used mostly for transradial amputations. A skin lined tunnel is made through the biceps and a rod is inserted through the tunnel that is attached by cable to the terminal device.
Ligatures	The process of binding or tying; sutures.
Myodesis	Attaching the ends of muscles to the end of the bone in amputation surgery.
Myoplasty	Attaching the cut ends of muscles over the end of a bone in amputation surgery.
Prosthesis	Artificial replacement of a body part.
Prosthetist	Individual who makes artificial limbs for the upper or lower extremities. A prosthetist who has completed a prescribed course of study and passed a certifying examination is allowed to use the initials "CP."
Reconstruction aides	Early physical therapists who joined the U.S. Army during World War I. After the war, these individuals came together and formed the American Physical Therapy Association.
Residual limb	The part of the limb that remains after amputation. It is also called the stump or residuum.
Septicemia	The presence of pathogenic organisms in the blood, leading to infection.

REFERENCES

1. Wilson, AB, Jr: History of amputation surgery and prosthetics. In Bowker, JH, and Michael, JW (eds.): Atlas of Limb Prosthetics: Surgical and Prosthetic Principles. Mosby-Year Book, St. Louis, 1992, pp. 3–16.
2. Garrison, FH: An Introduction to the History of Medicine. WB Saunders, Philadelphia, 1929.
3. Wilson, AB: Limb Prosthetics: 1970. Artificial Limbs 14:184–189, 1957.
4. Talbott, JH: A Biographical History of Medicine: Excerpts and Essays on the Men and Their Work. Grune & Stratton, New York, 1970.
5. Sanders, GT: Lower Limb Amputations: A Guide to Rehabilitation. FA Davis, Philadelphia, 1986.
6. Dederich, R: Technique of myoplastic amputations. Ann R Coll Surg Engl 40:222–227, 1967.
7. Burgess, E, Traub, JE, and Wilson, AB, Jr: Immediate postsurgical prosthetics in the managment of lower extremity amputees. Veterans Administration TR 10-5, U.S. Government Printing Office, Washington, DC, 1967.
8. Weiss, M: Myoplastic Amputation, Immediate Prosthesis and Early Ambulation. U.S. Depart-

ment of Health, Education, and Welfare, U.S. Government Printing Office, Washington, DC (no date given).

9. Sarmiento, A, May, BJ, Sinclair, WF, et al: Lower extremity amputation: The impact of immediate post surgical prosthetic fitting. Clin Orthop 68:22–31, 1970.

10. Most, RS, and Sinnock, P: The epidemiology of lower extremity amputations in diabetic individuals. Diabetes Care 6:87–91, 1983.

11. Schuch, CM, and Pritham, CH: International standards organization terminology: Application to prosthetics and orthotics. Journal of Prosthetics and Orthotics 6:29–33, 1994.

12. Sanders, R, and Helfet, D: The choice between limb salvage and amputation: Trauma. In Bowker, JH, and Michael, JW (eds.): Atlas of Limb Prosthetics: Surgical and Prosthetic Principles. Mosby-Year Book, St. Louis, 1992, pp 19–24.

13. Ouellette, EA, McAuliffe, JA, and Carneiro, R: Partial-hand amputation: Surgical principles. In Bowker, JH, and Michael, JW (eds.): Atlas of Limb Prosthetics: Surgical and Prosthetic Principles. Mosby-Year Book, St. Louis, 1992, pp 199–216.

14. May, BJ: A statewide amputee rehabilitation programme. Prosthet Orthot Int 2:24–26, 1978.

chapter two

Peripheral Vascular Diseases

OBJECTIVES

At the end of this chapter, all students are expected to:

1 Discuss the etiology and clinical features of major disorders of the peripheral vascular system that may lead to amputation.

2 Differentiate among chronic and acute arterial and venous diseases.

3 Discuss medical and surgical management of peripheral vascular diseases.

4 Discuss the functional effects of peripheral vascular diseases.

Physical therapy students are expected to:

5 Develop an assessment plan for an individual with peripheral vascular disease.

6 Interpret the results of a physical therapy assessment.

7 Develop a plan of care for an individual with peripheral vascular disease.

Arteriosclerosis causes most lower extremity amputation today. Physical therapists (PTs) and physical therapist assistants (PTAs) may treat an individual with an ulcerated foot from peripheral vascular disease; they may later treat the same person after lower extremity amputation. An individual with diabetes who undergoes one amputation for arteriosclerosis has a 51 percent chance of having a second amputation within 5 years.[1] As discussed in Chapter 5, care of the remaining extremity is an important part of the postamputation treatment program. The purpose of this chapter is to provide an overview of the peripheral vascular diseases that may lead to amputation or that may be present in individuals who have had an amputation. It is not meant to provide a complete study of all peripheral vascular diseases.

case studies

Diana Magnolia: a 54-year-old woman with a history of insulin dependent diabetes mellitus (IDDM) diagnosed 15 years ago. She is an outpatient referred for treatment of an ulcer on the plantar surface of the left first metatarsal head.

Benny Pearl: a 62-year-old man referred one day after right femoral/popliteal bypass for partial occlusion of the lower femoral artery.

Charley Johnson: a 59-year-old man referred for treatment of lower extremity edema and a stasis ulcer just proximal to the right medial malleolus.

CASE STUDY QUESTIONS

1 How would you diagnostically classify the condition of each of these people? Differentiate between arterial and venous disease and between acute and chronic vascular disease.

2 Describe the pathophysiology of each diagnosis, differentiating among major signs and symptoms. What additional information do you need before you can evaluate or treat each client? Supplement the information in this chapter with any pathophysiology reference.

3 What are the primary medical and surgical strategies used in the management of these diseases?

Physical Therapy Students:

4 For each client named, determine your course of action at this time. What data are needed to complete an evaluation? How would you prioritize the data? (Given a limited time, which data are critical to obtain early and which can be delayed?) What are the best sources of each datum (e.g., direct assessment, medical chart)? Justify your selection.

5 In your laboratory sessions, practice pertinent assessment activities. Role play each of the clients as accurately as possible. Do not look ahead to the next case study section until you have completed these items.

Pathophysiology and Etiology

Clients are rarely referred to physical therapy for preventive care in the early stages of peripheral vascular disease. However, clients with peripheral vascular disease may be referred for rehabilitation following total joint replacement or cerebral vascular accident. PTs and PTAs need to be alert to the early symptoms of arterial insufficiency and to teach proper foot care (see Chap. 3) Clients with severe vascular disease, such as the individuals described in the case studies, are referred for treatment. Prevention of further disability is an important part of the total management of vascular disease. The reader is encouraged to review the normal physiology of the vascular system as a point of reference in learning about vascular diseases.

ACUTE VASCULAR DISEASES

Venous Thrombosis

General anesthesia, immobilization, obesity, myocardial disease, venous disease, and cerebral vascular accidents are all risk factors for the formation of a thrombus in the superficial or deep venous system.[2] A clot or thrombus forms, often near a venous valve where venous blood may pool, and attaches to the vein wall. It grows quickly, blocking venous flow and leading to a pooling of blood behind the thrombus. The pressure stretches the venous walls, causing pain and inflammation.

The term **thrombophlebitis** refers to a thrombus in the superficial venous system.[3] Thrombi in the superficial veins are easily diagnosed and rarely become emboli. Edema is present around the site of the thrombus; the involved veins are raised, red, warm, and tender on palpation.

A thrombus in the deep vein system (a deep venous thrombosis or DVT) may become an embolus that is then pushed through the veins to the pulmonary system, possibly causing death. Most pulmonary emboli are believed to start as thrombi in the deep veins of the lower leg. Data on the incidence of pulmonary embolism are inconsistent because of difficulty in diagnosis; however, it is the fourth leading cause of sudden death in the United States.[4] DVT may lead to venous inflammation, valve damage, and chronic venous problems. Pain and tenderness in the calf, swelling of the lower leg, and redness following venous distribution have all been associated with a diagnosis of DVT; however, they are not reliable signs and are also associated with many other diagnoses.[5] Homans' sign, passive dorsiflexion of the ankle that causes pain in the calf or popliteal area, is likewise unreliable and nonspecific; approximately 50 percent of individuals with positive Homans' sign do not have DVT.[1] Venography, an invasive radiographic examination of the veins, is the most reliable test for DVT.

Cases of suspected DVT or superficial venous thrombus represent a medical emergency and should be reported to a physician for further evaluation. Therapy for acute DVT combines anticoagulant and thrombolytic drugs and bed rest with gradual exercises of the lower extremities to control edema. When ambulation is resumed, elastic stockings are used to control edema. Thrombophlebitis is also treated with anticoagulants; however, ambulation may be resumed earlier than with a DVT. Neither DVT nor thrombophlebitis leads to amputation.

Acute Arterial Occlusion

Acute arterial occlusion may result from trauma or embolus. The client reports acute pain in an area distal to the occlusion. On examination, the limb is pale and pulseless; the client describes it as cold and paralyzed. Acute arterial occlusion is a medical emergency because nerves and skeletal muscles tolerate ischemia for only 4 to 6 hours, whereas the skin tolerates ischemia for about 10 hours.[6] Diagnosis can be confirmed with Doppler ultrasound, a noninvasive measure of blood flow (Fig. 2.1). Doppler ultrasound is versatile and can be used to measure venous or arterial flow or to determine the status of venous valves. Briefly, the Doppler transmits a signal into the vessel and reflects back the sound waves of the movement of the blood through that vessel. It can detect pulses that might otherwise be inaudible and measure systolic blood pressure

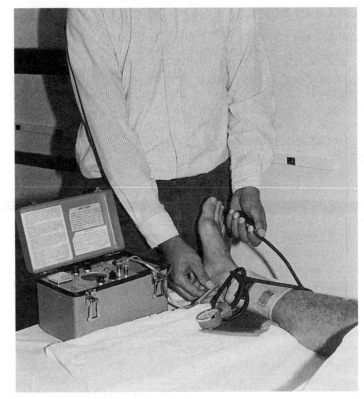

FIGURE 2.1
Doppler ultrasound may be used to measure blood flow, specifically, the ankle/brachial index (ABI).

accurately.[7] Doppler evaluation is discussed further later in this chapter. Treatment of an acute arterial occlusion varies with the severity of blockage. Anticoagulation therapy and thromboembolectomy may be performed. Suspected incidents of acute arterial occlusions must be referred immediately for medical evaluation and treatment or irreversible tissue ischemia and amputation may result.

CHRONIC VASCULAR DISEASES

Arteriosclerosis Obliterans

The term **arteriosclerosis obliterans (ASO)** refers to thickening, hardening, and narrowing of the walls of arteries.[8] Atherosclerosis is a form of ASO that affects the intima of large arteries; fibrous plaques narrow the vessels, eventually leading to ischemia. When related to diabetes, ASO tends to affect medium and small arteries of the lower extremities and is usually more rapidly progressive.

ASO occurs in about 5 percent of men over age 50 and women over age 60. About 25 percent of individuals with ASO eventually require reconstructive surgery and about 5 percent eventually require major amputation.[9] The number of cases increases when ASO is associated with diabetes. Approximately 15 percent of individuals with diabetes have ASO 15 years after onset; 45 percent have ASO 20 years after. Individuals with diabetes account for more than 50 percent of the amputations performed in the United States today.[1,10]

Chronic Venous Insufficiency

The term **chronic venous insufficiency** (CVI) describes a condition that may affect superficial or deep veins and is estimated to be statistically underreported. Varicose veins, a chronic problem of the superficial venous system, affect 1.5 to 5.2 percent of the population.[11,12] Insufficiency of the deep venous system is likewise not well reported in the literature, but venous ulcers are estimated to appear in about 1 percent of the population.[13] Although many of our clients may suffer from varicose veins, we rarely get involved unless the client has a venous ulcer or long standing edema from insufficiency of the deep venous system. Individuals with arterial insufficiency, particularly with diabetes, may also have CVI.

To understand the problems encountered in the development of venous ulcers, normal venous physiology must be understood. Deep veins and calf muscles pump the blood toward the heart during the systolic phase of venous contraction. Valves in the perforating veins prevent retrograde flow. During the diastolic (relaxation) phase, the calf veins refill as blood flows from the superficial to the deep veins through the perforating veins. Venous pressure is higher in the deep veins during the contracting (systolic) phase and higher in the superficial veins during the relaxing (diastolic) phase. Damage to the valves of the perforating veins affects the systolic phase. Incompetent valves allow blood to flow from the deep to the superficial system, thus increasing pressure in the deep system. Venous occlusions contribute to the increased pressure, as does the effect of gravity in the upright position. The greater the hydrostatic pressure in the superficial system during the systolic phase, the less blood is pumped out of the deep system toward the heart. Over time, venous capillaries proliferate. Increased capillary permeability allows fluid, rich in fibrins and other materials, to leak into the interstitial space, creating the characteristic edema associated with CVI. To manage the edematous limb, it is important to differentiate between edema secondary to venous insufficiency and edema secondary to lymphatic disease. Table 2.1 compares arterial and venous diseases.

Thromboangiitis Obliterans (Buerger's Disease)

Thromboangiitis obliterans (TAO) is an inflammation of small and medium sized arteries and veins that occurs in a very small percentage of the population. TAO, also called Buerger's disease after the physician who first identified it, starts distally and progresses proximally, involving both upper and lower extremities. It is initially diagnosed in young men who smoke, although the incidence of the disease in women has grown in the past decades, probably because of improved diagnosis. Etiologically, it is directly related to smoking. It is exacerbated by smoking and improves when the client stops. Symptoms include bilateral intermittent claudication starting distally, possible superficial phlebitis, and decreased tolerance of cold in the hands and fingers. Clients may experience repeated episodes of pedal claudication and phlebitis. The major

T A B L E   2 . 1   **PERIPHERAL VASCULAR DISEASES**

Disease	Etiology	Pathology	Major Symptoms
Arteriosclerosis obliterans (ASO) without diabetes	More men than women; over age 50; risk factors include smoking, obesity, hypertension, hyperlipidemia, sedentary lifestyle	Large artery occlusive disease; affects intima of arteries with luminal narrowing; fibrous plaques develop, associated with hypertension and coronary artery disease	Intermittent claudication, then rest; pain relieved by standing; absent or decreased pedal pulses; dry skin in lower leg; clubbing of toenails; hair loss on lower leg; ischemia of toes, ulcer on weight-bearing foot surface
Arteriosclerosis with diabetes	Over age 40; risk factors same as ASO without diabetes; affects lower extremities more than upper extremities	Medium and small arteries involved; fatty streaks lead to fibrous plaques and narrowing of arteries	Same as ASO without diabetes plus decreased or absent sensation of the foot; renal complications; impaired vision; loss of muscle strength in distal segments
Chronic venous insufficiency (CVI)	Affects about 1% of population; superficial and deep veins may be involved; incidence increases with age	Blood flows back to superficial veins; secondary to damaged perforating valves; leads to increased pressure and decreased flow back to heart; new venous capillaries and increased fibrinolytic buildup prevent normal exchange and lead to cell death	Edema (pitting early, hard later); dilated veins; leg pain (heaviness, ache while standing relieved by elevation); cutaneous changes (brownish color, dermatitis); skin ulcers above medial malleolus
Thromboangiitis obliterans (TAO)	Men 20–40 years of age; tobacco users; incidence 12/100,000 population	Vasospastic and arteriosclerosis components affecting small and medium arteries and veins of upper and lower extremities; starts distally; progresses proximally	Bilateral ischemia that starts distally and leads to ulceration and amputation; superficial phlebitis and dyesthesia; may have rubor or cyanosis; pedal claudication; rest pain

treatment is the cessation of all tobacco use. A small number of individuals with TAO who do not stop smoking may require amputation of one or more distal limbs. These individuals represent a very small percentage of individuals requiring amputation for vascular disease.[14]

Diagnosis and Assessment

DIAGNOSIS OF ARTERIOSCLEROSIS OBLITERANS

Age, sex, hypertension, diabetes, elevated serum cholesterol concentrations and low density lipid (LDL) levels in the blood, obesity, smoking, and sedentary lifestyle are all risk factors that have been associated with arteriosclerosis obliterans (ASO). Smoking doubles the risk of ASO in both men and women; hypertension triples the risk.[15–17] The initial diagnosis is frequently made by the family practitioner, and clients are not seen by a vascular specialist until the disease is fairly well advanced.

Intermittent claudication is often the first symptom that leads the client to seek medical attention. Intermittent claudication is a cramping calf pain that occurs on walking until ischemia of the muscles of the lower leg is present. As the disease progresses, the distance that the client is able to walk becomes shorter and shorter before claudication occurs. Severe ASO is characterized by rest pain, a cramping or aching pain in the calf or foot that occurs during sleep. Clients get up in the night to put the limb in a dependent position and may eventually opt to sleep in a sitting position. Some edema of the lower leg may result from maintaining the limb in a dependent position for prolonged periods. Rest pain occurs in about 24 percent of individuals experiencing intermittent claudication.[9] Severe ischemia may lead to foot ulcers. Two types of ulcers are related to arterial insufficiency. Individuals with large vessel disease not associated with diabetes and with severe ischemia and rest pain may develop ulcers at the end of a toe or between two toes. These ulcers are caused by ischemic necrosis and dry gangrene. Ulcers may also occur secondary to minor trauma or pressure on the feet. Although they are more common among individuals with diabetes, they may also occur in those with severe ischemia of the lower extremities. About 5 percent of individuals who have intermittent claudication sustain a lower extremity amputation secondary to gangrene of the foot.[9] Foot ulcers, a major problem among individuals with ASO and diabetes, are discussed in more detail in Chapter 3.

MEDICAL ASSESSMENT OF ARTERIOSCLEROSIS OBLITERANS

The physician usually diagnoses ASO by history and physical examination. One should compare one limb with the other because one side is frequently more involved. Palpation of the femoral, popliteal, posterior tibial, and dorsalis pedis pulses helps to pinpoint areas of diminished circulation. Inadequate circulation may also lead to dependent rubor; the limb is elevated at an angle about 60 degrees for 1 minute, then placed in a dependent position. If the limb turns red, this is a rebound from the period of hypoxia and an indication of dysvascularity. A walking test may also be performed, with the observer noting how far a client can walk on a treadmill before developing intermittent claudication.

Laboratory tests may include Doppler ankle/brachial index (ABI), segmental volume plethysmography, duplex ultrasonography, magnetic resonance imaging (MRI), or arteriography. The ABI test is easy to perform and quite reliable. Ankle and brachial systolic measures are obtained by inflating a blood pressure cuff above systolic pressure and determining when the resumption of flow oc-

T A B L E 2 . 2   **IMPLICATIONS OF ANKLE BRACHIAL INDEX READINGS**

ABI Reading	Indication
0.9 to 1.3	Normal reading
0.4 to 0.9	Intermittent claudication present
0.25 to 0.4	Rest pain present
Below 0.25	Ulcers and gangrene

curs by placing the Doppler probe over the radial artery in the arm and over the tibial or dorsalis pedis arteries in the ankle. The ratio is obtained by dividing the ankle systolic pressure by the brachial systolic pressure. Normal readings range from 0.9 to 1.3 while a reading below 0.9 indicates a degree of arterial insufficiency. Table 2.2 indicates the implications of ranges of results.

Segmental volume plethysmography combines measures of segmental systolic pressure taken at the thigh, calf, and ankle, with assessment of pulse volume wave forms that accurately reflect vascular status.[9]

Transcutaneous oxygen measurements (TC PO_2) assess tissue metabolism as a function of perfusion by reflecting the percentage of oxygen, and thus circulation, in the tissues. It may be used to predict the healing potential for an ulcer or amputation.

MRI provides the physician with an accurate estimate of blood flow velocity using a noninvasive method. The limited resolution of small peripheral arteries and its high cost limits the use of MRI in the evaluation of peripheral arterial disease.

The use of arteriography, an invasive technique where dye is injected into an artery and then followed by radiographs, has decreased with the advent of reliable noninvasive techniques. Arteriography is usually performed before reconstructive surgery.

PHYSICAL THERAPY ASSESSMENT OF ARTERIOSCLEROSIS OBLITERANS

History and Interview

The PT should obtain a detailed history and perform a careful physical examination to document the extent of vascular insufficiency. Information needed in the interview includes other medical problems, medications, lifestyle, and the client's perception of the symptoms.

The PT and PTA need to know if the client has related diseases such as hypertension and cardiac disease. Having clients describe their medical problems provides some insight into the clients' understanding of associated diseases.

The PT and PTA should obtain a list of current medications to assess their possible effects on therapeutic activities. Anticoagulants make the client more prone to bruising or bleeding. Hypertension is controlled by various drugs including diuretics, beta blockers, and angiotensin converting enzyme (ACE) inhibitors. Diuretics may cause frequent urination. Beta blockers may limit exercise tolerance with clients complaining of dizziness and weakness if overstressed. ACE inhibitors may also cause dizziness and a sense of weakness in some cases. The problem of drug reactions and interactions is complex; clients may be taking several prescription drugs provided by different physicians and may also be taking over the counter medications. Some of the medications may interfere with, rather than enhance, function. Drug reactions must be suspected when client complaints or behaviors are not obviously related. Carrying a small up to date pharmacology reference book is recommended.

Information regarding current lifestyle is valuable to set realistic treatment goals and to encourage compliance in home activities. What is the client's job? What are the demands at home? Does he or she have recreational activities? Is the client a smoker? If yes, how much does he or she smoke? Does the client follow an appropriate diet? Although the client probably knows the negative effects of smoking and a diet high in cholesterol and salt, the PT and PTA can support and encourage necessary lifestyle changes.

Asking the client to describe current symptoms provides information on the client's perceptions. What are the current symptoms? When and how often do they occur? What is the intensity? What makes them worse or better?

Physical Assessment

Skin condition, color, presence or absence of hair, and condition of toenails must be noted. Individuals with arterial insufficiency often have dry, scaly skin, no hair, and thick toenails (Fig. 2.2). Toes may be clubbed. Skin temperature is not a good indicator of arterial insufficiency because many conditions, several of them benign, contribute to cold skin. The presence or absence of lower extremity pulses is noted. Collateral circulation, developed over time, may pro-

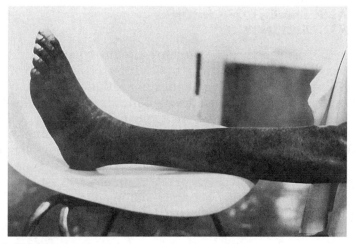

FIGURE 2.2
Leg showing arterial dysvascularity.

vide adequate circulation to the lower extremity even in the absence of pulses in the major vessels.

If the client has a skin ulcer, record the size, location, amount and color of drainage, and depth. There are various ways to document wound size; commercially available grids on acetate or sterile x ray film can be put over the wound and traced or photographed. The depth of the wound can be measured with a sterile cotton tipped applicator.[18] Sterile techniques should be used when measuring an ulcer.

Although edema is more often associated with CVI, clients with ASO may have edema related to local inflammation, associated venous disease, congestive heart disease, renal or kidney problems, or the prolonged dependent position of a limb. Edema is easily documented by taking circumferential girth measurements at regular and documented intervals. Edema, particularly in the foot, can also be measured with a volumeter. The volumeter is filled with water, the foot is placed in the plexiglas device, and the displaced water is collected in a graduated cylinder. Both limbs should be measured for comparison.

Clients with diabetes frequently exhibit decreased sensation in the foot and ankle, and possibly in the lower leg. Light touch and differentiation of sharp and dull pressure are the most important sensory tests to perform. Proprioception and vibratory sense may also be impaired.

Inactivity, edema, and musculoskeletal changes may decrease range of motion of the toes and foot that, in turn, may affect pressures generated in the shoe during ambulation. Careful goniometric measurement of all ranges of ankle motion and strength determination of the foot and ankle is an important part of the evaluation. These parameters of both lower extremities indicate the client's functional level for mobility.

Many individuals do not wear properly fitted shoes; careful assessment of the client's footwear is part of the basic assessment of any individual with vascular disease. Some people cannot afford proper shoes. Medicare, at this time, does not provide reimbursement for regular shoes for individuals with severe vascular disease. Foot problems and protective shoes are explored in greater detail in Chapter 3.

MEDICAL ASSESSMENT OF CHRONIC VENOUS INSUFFICIENCY

Chronic venous disease is classified into three grades (Table 2.3). The cause of venous ulcers, a characteristic of Grade III, has not been well defined. Browse and Burnand[19] suggest that venous ulceration is related to the proliferation of venous capillaries and the increased fibrins in the fluid leaking into the interstitial space. Venous ulcers are characteristically found just proximal to the medial malleolus, where the lower three major perforating veins are located and the greatest hydrostatic pressure is concentrated when the person is in the upright position. Fluid leakage into the interstitial tissues is probably greatest in this area. Before the development of an ulcer, the skin usually becomes dark brown, subcutaneous fat becomes indurated, and dermatitis and evidence of inflammation as well as edema may be seen. Venous ulcers are shallow and weepy with ill defined borders.[13,20]

In contrast venography, dye is injected into the vein and radiographs are taken of the limb. This is the most accurate method of evaluating the veins.

T A B L E 2 . 3 **CHRONIC VENOUS INSUFFICIENCY CLASSIFICATION**

Grade	Symptoms
I	Mild episodes of edema during upright activity that resolve easily with rest and limb elevation
	Edema limited to the foot and possibly the ankle and usually less than 1 centimeter
	No changes in skin condition or pigmentation
II	Varicosities may be observable
	Edema in foot and ankle greater than 1 centimeter that may not resolve with limb elevation
	Client complains of heavy aching sensation with prolonged standing
	Evidence of beginning changes in pigmentation in lower leg
	Beginning induration of the skin
III	Severe thick edema extending to midcalf
	Client complains of heavy aching pain after short periods of standing
	Dark brown pigmentation in the lower leg and ankle
	Evidence of skin induration, dermatitis, and eczema of the lower leg
	Weeping, shallow ulcer proximal to the medial malleolus

However, noninvasive tests, including the multilevel tourniquet test, plethysmography, Doppler assessment, and duplex imaging, are almost as accurate. The multilevel tourniquet test involves placing tourniquets in the upper and lower thigh, upper calf, and above the malleoli with the client in the supine position. The client then stands and the tourniquets are removed, starting at the bottom. Superficial and deep vein competence is determined by the degree of filling of the lesser and greater saphenous veins.[13]

There are two major types of plethysmography, which measures blood flow. Impedance plethysmography uses changes in voltage generated by blood flow as a reflection of volume. Air plethymosgraphy records graphically the length of time it takes for a vein to refill after its flow is cut off by a pneumatic cuff placed proximally on the limb.

Doppler imaging has been described previously. The Doppler sound head is placed over the vein being evaluated while the examiner squeezes the limb proximally. Changes in the flow sound reflect valve function. If the valves are functioning properly, there should be no increase in blood flow. Physical therapists can use small portable Doppler machines for arterial or venous evaluation.[7,13,21]

Duplex ultrasound imaging provides a computerized image of the superficial and deep veins and the perforating system generated by ultrasound waves. It also images the arterial system, making it a flexible evaluation tool for the physician.[22,23]

PHYSICAL THERAPY ASSESSMENT OF CHRONIC VENOUS INSUFFICIENCY

Clients with CVI may be referred to physical therapy for treatment of edema. As with arterial insufficiency, the assessment includes taking a careful history and making a thorough physical examination. It is important to know if the edema is relieved overnight, if the client wears elastic stockings, and if the client is able to elevate the legs during the day. Circumferential limb measurements provide objective data for determining the effects of treatment. Measurements are taken at regular intervals (usually every 2.5 to 4 centimeters) for the entire limb segment (Fig. 2.3). Bony landmarks are used as reference points for each measurement (e.g., 4 centimeters above the medial malleolus). Foot measurements need to be taken as well, usually around the head of the metatarsals, at a measured midpoint of the foot, and around the heel at the most distal point.

Although edema usually does not interfere with strength, it may limit the range of ankle motion so that goniometric measurements are necessary. The condition of the skin must be noted and the presence of ulceration documented. It is valuable to inspect the client's shoes. Foot edema causes many clients to wear slippers or other loose fitting shoes that may hamper gait and fail to protect the foot from injury. Pain is assessed in terms of severity and when it occurs. Venous pain must be differentiated from arterial pain. Pain associated with CVI occurs after prolonged standing and is reported as a dull ache and heaviness in the lower leg. It is relieved by elevation of the legs. In contrast, arterial insufficiency is a sharp, cramping pain of the calf. It occurs either at night or with walking. As with all clients, information on the person's understanding of the disease process, lifestyle demands, and expectations are a necessary part of the evaluation.

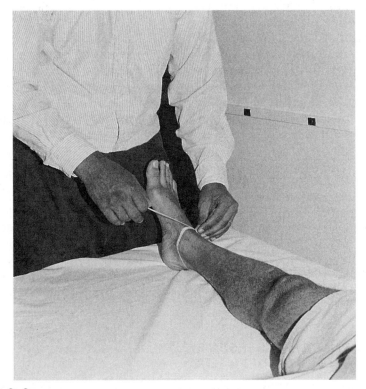

FIGURE 2.3
Taking circumferential measurements of a leg.

case studies

Figures 2.4, 2.5, and 2.6 are the physical therapy assessments for Diana Magnolia, Benny Pearl, and Charley Johnson. Refer to them when answering the following questions.

HISTORY:
IDDM diagnosed 19 years ago; has always been poorly controlled; height 5'6"; weight 210 lb.

SOCIAL:
Ms. Magnolia is a waitress who lives in a rural town with two of her grown children. She spends a great deal of time on her feet. She has no hobbies. She has medical insurance (not Major Medical, however) through her employment.

PHYSICAL:

Skin:
Decreased sensation in both feet; normal sensation throughout the rest of the lower extremities. Both lower extremities are relatively hairless from about mid calf down. The skin of the right leg is shiny particularly in the distal 3rd of the lower leg. The nail of the right great toe is thickened and discolored. Pedal pulses bilaterally are absent. Both feet are cool to touch. Ulcer on L foot is 2.5 cm diameter; relatively shallow; no evidence of granulous tissue and no drainage. The tissue around the ulcer is white and callused. The tissue within the ulcer is pinkish red. She has had the ulcer for about 6 weeks.

Range of Motion:
Left ankle: plantar flexion: active=0–20 deg; passive=0–25 deg; dorsiflexion: active=0 deg of neutral; passive = 5 deg; inversion & eversion: active = 0–5 deg; passive = 0–10 deg.
Left knee and hip within normal limits active and passive.
Right ankle: plantar flexion: active and passive= 0–25 degrees; dorsiflexion: active and passive= 0–5 degrees; inversion & eversion active and passive=0–10 degrees.
Right hip and knee are within normal limits active and passive.

Edema:
No differences in girth noted between the lower extremities.

Muscle Strength:
Left lower extremity dorsi= Fair (3/5); Plantar Flexion = Fair+ (3+/5); Eversion/inversion = Poor+(2+/5). Right lower extremity ankle musculature is Good (4/5). Rest of the musculature of both lower extremities is within normal limits. General body strength appears to be within normal limits.

Pain:
Denies pain in the ulcer area. Cramping pain in the arch of her left foot interferes with walking long distances. Occasional cramping pain at night.

GENERAL INFORMATION:
Patient walks without external support. Wears old loafers and socks on both feet. A gauze pad covers the ulcer. No gait deviations. Patient states she controls her diabetes with daily injection of insulin and is taking Lasix for control of high blood pressure. She denies any other medication. Ms. Magnolia states she is independent in self care activities. Ms. Magnolia states she does not drink alcohol, but smokes about a pack a day. She has no previous history of ulcers. She has been treated for high blood pressure for about 4 years. She is being followed in the eye clinic for early developing cataracts.

FIGURE 2.4
Physical therapy evaluation for Diana Magnolia.

HISTORY:
Prior to surgery Right ankle-brachial Doppler index was .4; segmental plethysmography indicated a significant obstruction between the upper and lower thigh. Arteriography showed a complete occlusion of the superficial femoral artery with fair collateral flow below the occlusion. History of COPD, CAD. Prior to surgery, he was unable to walk more than 10 meters before having pain in the right calf and foot.

SOCIAL:
Mr. Pearl and his wife live in a small frame house on the outskirts of town. They have 3 grown children in other parts of the country. Mr. Pearl owns and operates a service station in town. Mrs. Pearl works part-time as an LPN in a nearby hospital. In the months before surgery he found it increasingly difficult to walk and work.

PHYSICAL:
The physical examination was somewhat difficult to perform since Mr. Pearl had some difficulty following instructions and seemed a bit confused. Findings are subject to reevaluation at a later date.

Vitals: BP 145/95; respiration 16; pulse 90 at the beginning of the evaluation.

Skin:
Appears to have relatively normal sensation throughout both lower extremities. Both legs have little hair, skin is normal in appearance and warm. There is a dressing in the anterior groin area extending to the medial thigh on the right and the sutures are in place. There is no draining from the incisions.

Edema:
No evidence of edema in the lower extremities.

Range of Motion:
On gross evaluation, the left lower extremity appears actively and passively within normal limits. Range of ankle motion is grossly within normal limits. Mr. Pearl can move the right leg but full ROM testing was delayed.

Muscle Strength:
Muscle strength of the left lower extremity was grossly within normal limits. Muscle testing on the right was delayed secondary to surgery and the risk of stressing the incision. Mr. Pearl can tolerate manual resistance for ankle motions.

Pain:
Pain reported at the incision site is 4 on 0–10 scale. Mr. Pearl is afraid the bypass won't work.

Functional:
Mr. Pearl appears a little confused and is not a clear historian. Chart review indicates that he has not stood since surgery and cannot get from bed to chair by himself. He was able to turn from left side to back in bed. Mr. Pearl needed moderate physical help from the therapist to transfer in and out of bed into the wheelchair and step by step cueing. He put minimal weight on his right leg, was hesitant to try to help himself and was slow in following directions. He made minimal attempts to wheel the chair himself despite encouragement. He appeared to tire quickly and said he wanted to go back to bed.

MEDICATION:
Procardia, Coumadin, Capoten, Darvocet and Lasix.

GENERAL INFORMATION:
Smokes about 2 packs day.

FIGURE 2.5
Physical therapy evaluation for Benny Pearl.

HISTORY:
Mr. Johnson reports having had varicose veins and venous problems for many years.

SOCIAL:
Mr. Johnson is a textile worker who has been referred because he can no longer spend a full day standing at his machine. He is currently on sick leave from his job. He has 2 weeks of sick leave credit left. He is covered by a Blue Cross/Blue Shield policy through his plant. Mr. Johnson is married with 6 children ranging in age from 17 to 39; two are living at home. His wife also works at the textile mill and the 17 year old daughter works after school and on weekends at Smith Drugs. The Johnsons live in a small wooden house which they own. Mr. Johnson used to work weekends as a security guard but had to stop about a month ago because of his legs.

PHYSICAL:
5'7" tall; weighs 185 lb.
Skin:
Right Lower Extremity: Area approximately 9.5 cm long and 6 cm wide is red, weeping, and beginning to give evidence of ulceration. Dark purplish brown ring about 4 cm wide around the ulceration which is covered with a thickened, desensitized skin. Decreased sensation all around the lower leg and proximal foot. Sensation around the toes and knee appears relatively normal. No hair on the right lower extremity below the knee.

Edema:
Edema evident in both lower extremities greater on the right. Right ankle around malleoli= 30.5 cm, L= 28 cm; 2" above medial malleoli = 32 cm both sides; circumference around head of metatarsals: Right = 31.5 cm; Left = 29 cm.

Left Lower Extremity: Some discoloration just above the medial malleoli with decreased sensation. Sensation is relatively normal around the toes and knee. No hair below the knee. When the patient stands for several minutes, the skin of both lower legs around the ankles and feet becomes a deeper purple.

Range of Motion:
All ranges of motion of both lower extremities are within normal limits except as follows: (active and passive ranges are the same)

	Left	Right
Dorsiflexion active & passive	0–9	0–3
Plantar flexion active & passive	0–15	0–10
Eversion active & passive	0–5	0–5
Inversion active & passive	0–10	0–5

Muscle Strength:
Musculature around both ankles is in the Fair+ (3+/5) range; rest of the lower extremity is in the Good to Good+ range (4+/5). Upper extremity strength appears to be within normal limits.

Pain:
Pain in the right lower extremity after standing for 15–20 minutes. Some pain in the left lower extremity but not as severe. Discolored areas in both legs itch frequently and severely. The itching is temporarily relieved by elevating the legs or soaking the feet in cold water.

GENERAL INFORMATION:
Mr. Johnson denies smoking or drinking alcoholic beverages. He states that he is independent in all self care activities. He walked into the department using a cane in his right hand and taking a shorter step with the right leg. He is wearing black slippers and black socks.

FIGURE 2.6
Physical therapy evaluation for Charley Johnson.

CASE STUDY ACTIVITIES

1 Write long and short term goals for each client on the basis of the information provided.
2 Develop a treatment plan for each client.
3 In the laboratory session, practice any evaluation or treatment procedure with which you are not familiar.

Management

MEDICAL AND PHYSICAL THERAPY MANAGEMENT OF ARTERIAL DISEASE

Improvement of arterial circulation is the major goal of medical and surgical management. Surgical interventions used to improve peripheral circulation include reconstruction such as femoropopliteal bypass, balloon angioplasty, and endarterectomy. The greater saphenous vein, reversed to prevent interference with blood flow by the valves, is generally used for femoropopliteal bypasses, although synthetic conduits may also be used. Balloon angioplasty involves the insertion of a catheter with a balloon tip inflated to the appropriate level to stretch and open the artery as it passes through. Endarterectomy involves removing some of the plaque that has accumulated inside an artery. A longitudinal study in Maryland in 1988 and 1989 revealed that, of 7210 procedures performed for peripheral arterial disease, 1185 were angioplasties, 4005 were bypasses, and 1890 were amputations.[24] Individuals treated initially by revascularization procedures tended to be white men under age 74 and with Medicare or private insurance. The incidence of diabetes and hypertension, positively related to the likelihood of amputation, was significantly greater in African Americans.[24] Individuals undergoing revascularization procedures are not routinely referred to physical therapy.

The major goals of physical therapy are to promote healing of any ulcer or wound, to prevent further injury, and to educate the client in the proper care of the extremities and in methods to enhance development of collateral circulation. Deficiencies in strength or range of motion must be addressed. See Chapter 3 for details of wound and ulcer care. Education is an important part of the care of individuals with peripheral vascular disease. Table 2.4 outlines aspects of the client education program. Long term care includes promoting the development of collateral circulation through an active exercise program. Walking is excellent for individuals with arterial insufficiency. They can increase their ambulatory capabilities by walking to the point of intermittent claudication, stopping until the cramp ceases, then walking again.[25–28] For individuals with active ulcers on limited weight bearing, a program of active exercises can be substituted.

MEDICAL AND PHYSICAL THERAPY MANAGEMENT OF VENOUS DISEASE

The primary goal in the medical and physical therapy management of CVI is to control venous hypertension and reduce edema. Education in proper skin care and in methods of preventing development or recurrence of ulcers is essential. The desired outcome of treatment is not only the healing of the existing ulcer

T A B L E 2.4 **CLIENT EDUCATION PROGRAMS**

Category	Arteriosclerosis	Venous Insufficiency
Disease process	Pathophysiology in simple terms; general prognosis; how pathology can be improved; what can increase problems; answer specific questions	
Foot and leg care	Keep feet and legs clean and dry; apply water absorbing lotion on dry skin, particularly after baths; check feet daily for pressure areas; wear supportive shoes; do not walk barefoot or with open shoes; keep full range of motion in feet and ankles; trim toenails straight across and guard against injury; obtain professional help for problem nails	Ankle pumps and toe motions for edema control; elevate feet and legs regularly; wear support stockings if prescribed; use water absorbing lotion on dry skin; do not use alcohol on skin; do not scratch irritated skin; watch for ulcer development
Pain management	For intermittent claudication: start a walking or bicycling program; exercise to the point of cramping, stop and rest a moment, then resume; exercise regularly, gradually increasing time or distance; for rest pain: elevate head of bed; wear socks to bed; no heating pads on legs, but can apply low heat to abdomen	Wear support stocking when out of bed; stop and do ankle pumps with legs at level of heart several times a day; when sitting, keep legs elevated about the level of heart; raise foot of bed.
Lifestyle	Discuss smoking, nutrition, stress, activity level; help client identify problem areas and find solutions	Discuss edema control, effects on prolonged standing, effects of air temperature, use of support stockings; help client identify problem areas and find solutions

but the prevention of new ulcers.[10] CVI cannot be cured, and therefore lifestyle changes are necessary for effective management.

The major treatment modality of the venous ulcer is compression through semirigid dressings, elastic stockings or wraps, or intermittent compression. Compression is believed to reduce venous hypertension by blocking transcapillary flow during contraction, thereby increasing the flow out of the deep veins. The amount of pressure needed to achieve such reduction increases with the severity of the disease. Semirigid dressings such as Unna's boot (a zinc impregnated semiocclusive dressing manufactured by Miles Pharmaceutical) provide wound care and compression at the same time. The rigid dressing helps protect the limb from injury. The disadvantages are the need for frequent reapplication by a health care professional, potential problems of personal hygiene, and occasional reactions to the medication. Standard postsurgical stockings offer uniform elastic compression from foot to knee or upper thigh; there are also individually constructed elastic stockings that provide graded compression.

Knee high custom made elastic stockings have been shown to be effective in the treatment of CVI.[12,29] Thigh high stockings may bind in the popliteal area and are difficult to keep in place. Most clients require compression at the ankle level but rarely above the knee. Clients should be given two pairs of stockings that should be replaced whenever they lose their elasticity. Clients need to be taught proper donning procedures and care of the stockings. Companies that manufacture the stockings generally provide care information to the client. If an ulcer is present, a dressing under the stocking provides extra compression to the area and keeps the stocking relatively clean. PTs and PTAs use kits (available from the manufacturers) to measure an individual for compression stockings. The limb needs to be measured after attempts to reduce edema through intermittent compression and elevation.

Elastic stockings are difficult to put on; many elderly people, particularly those with limited hand function, find it impossible to don the stockings properly. Elastic bandages can be substituted, although they are not as effective. While easier to apply, the elastic bandage loses its elasticity quickly, needs to be wrapped properly to provide appropriate pressure, must be rewrapped frequently, and occupies more space in the shoe than a stocking. Elastic bandages need to be applied starting with the toes and following a figure of eight pattern up the leg to just below the popliteal area. Overlapping the edges by at least 1 inch helps prevent exposed skin as the wrap changes position with client activity. For most clients, two 10 centimeter (4 inch) bandages are needed. Compliance with the use of elastic wraps is usually poor.

Proper skin care is important for individuals with venous disease as well as for those with arterial insufficiency. Water soluble lotion is recommended; it will not stain elastic stockings and usually feels more comfortable to the client.

Standing, walking, or sitting for prolonged periods contributes to edema. Clients need to sit or lie frequently with the legs elevated to about heart level. Although elevation to 45 or 50 degrees is advisable for the management of edema secondary to lymphatic disease, it is not recommended for CVI because it places too much stress on an already compromised system.

Intermittent compression is an effective tool to reduce edema (Fig. 2.7). Intermittent or sequential pumps may be used. The limb is covered with stockinet before insertion in the inflatable sleeve. Any ulcer must be covered with a plastic bag. The client needs to be comfortably placed in the supine position. Pressure is set to no more than 20 mmHg less than diastolic; settings as low as 40 mmHg have been found effective.[19] No available studies outline the effectiveness of any given on and off ratio. Generally 60 seconds on and 30 seconds off are used, although McCulloch and Hovde[20] recommend 90 seconds on and 30 seconds off. Treatments last generally 1 hour or longer. Small home units are available for home use.

Active ankle exercises are an important adjunct to the rest of the program. Muscle contraction contributes to pumping blood toward the heart in the deep venous system. The client is taught to perform flexion, extension, and circumduction of the ankle slowly through the full range of motion several times a day, particularly when supine. General active exercises, including walking, are not contraindicated and may be beneficial. The client should wear elastic stockings at all times when exercising, and may need to spend some time supine after exercise to prevent or control edema.

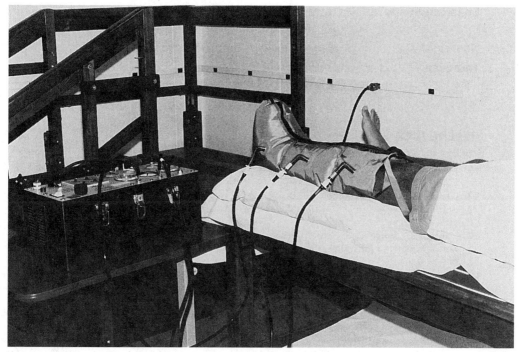

FIGURE 2.7
Applying intermittent compression to a leg.

SUMMARY

Most clients treated for major amputations of the lower limb have some form of vascular disease. Although CVI is not a primary cause of amputation, individuals with arterial disease may also have venous insufficiency. PTs and PTAs must integrate the care of the vascular disease and the remaining extremity into the total care of the individual with a lower extremity amputation.

GLOSSARY

Arteriosclerosis	Thickening, hardening, and narrowing of the walls of the arteries.
Atherosclerosis	A form of arteriosclerosis in which plaques composed of lipids and other materials form on the intima of the arteries.
Doppler ultrasound	A noninvasive method of detecting changes in blood flow through an artery.
Embolus	A clot or mass of foreign materials that obstructs a vein or artery. An embolus may be a part of a thrombus that has broken off and traveled to a vessel too small to allow passage.

Endarterectomy	Surgical removal of the lining of an artery. May be performed on major arteries to increase blood flow.
Neuropathy	Any disease of the nervous system.
Thrombus	A clot made of blood and other materials that forms and attaches to the walls of an artery or vein.

REFERENCES

1. Most, RS, and Sinnock, P: The epidemiology of lower extremity amputations in diabetic individuals. Diabetes Care 6:87–91, 1983.
2. Graor, RA, and Bartholomew, JR: Deep vein thrombosis. In Young, JR, Graor, RA, Olin, JW, and Bartholomew, JR (eds.): Peripheral Vascular Diseases. Mosby-Year Book, St. Louis, 1991, pp 403–422.
3. Young, JR: Clinical clues to peripheral vascular disease. In Young, JR, Graor, RA, Olin, JW, and Bartholomew, JR (eds.) Peripheral Vascular Diseases. Mosby-Year Book, St. Louis, 1991, pp 3–20.
4. Graor, RA, and Bartholomew, JR: Pulmonary embolism. In Young, JR, Graor, RA, Olin, JW, and Bartholomew, JR (eds.): Peripheral Vascular Diseases. Mosby-Year Book, St. Louis, 1991, pp 423–442.
5. Hull, RD, Hirsh, J, Sackett, DL, et al: Clinical validity of a negative venogram in patients with clinically suspected venous thrombosis. Circulation 64:622, 1981.
6. Comerota, AJ, and Leefmans, E: Acute arterial occlusions. In Young, JR, Graor, RA, Olin, JW, and Bartholomew, JR (eds.): Peripheral Vascular Diseases. Mosby-Year Book, St. Louis, 1991, pp 227–240.
7. MacKinnon, J: Doppler ultrasound assessment in peripheral vascular disease. In Kloth, LC, McCulloch, JM, and Feedar, JA (eds.): Wound Healing: Alternatives in Management. FA Davis, Philadelphia, 1990, pp 119–131.
8. Taber's Cyclopedic Medical Dictionary, ed 16. FA Davis, Philadelphia, 1989.
9. Krajewski, LP, and Olin, JW: Atherosclerosis of the aorta and lower extremities arteries. In Young, JR, Graor, RA, Olin, JW, and Bartholomew, JR (eds.): Peripheral Vascular Diseases. Mosby-Year Book, St. Louis, 1991, pp 179–200.
10. Reiber, GE, Pecoraro, RE, and Koepsell, TD: Risk factors for amputation in patients with diabetes mellitus: A case-control study. Ann. Intern Med 117:97–105, 1992.
11. Browse, NL, Burnand, KG, and Lea, TM (eds.): Diseases of the Veins: Pathology, Diagnosis and Treatment. Edward Arnold, London, 1988.
12. Widmer, LK: Peripheral venous disorders: Prevalence and sociomedical importance—observations in 4529 apparently healthy persons, Basic III Study. Bern, Hans Huber, 1978.
13. O'Donnell, TF, Jr: Chronic venous insufficiency and varicose veins. In Young, JR, Graor, RA, Olin, JW, and Bartholomew, JR (eds.): Peripheral Vascular Diseases. Mosby-Year Book, St. Louis, 1991, pp 443–482.
14. Joyce, JW: Thomboangiitis obliterans (Buerger's disease). In Young, JR, Graor, RA, Olin, JW, and Bartholomew, JR (eds.): Peripheral Vascular Diseases. Mosby-Year Book, St. Louis, 1991, pp 331–338.
15. Kannel, WB, and McGee, DL: Update on some epidemiologic features of intermittent claudication: The Framingham study. J Am Geriatr Soc 33:13, 1985.
16. Fowkes, FG, Housley, E, Riemersma, RA, et al: Smoking, lipids, glucose intolerance, and blood pressure as risk factors for peripheral atherosclerosis compared with ischemic heart disease in the Edinburgh Artery Study. Am J Epidemiol 135:331–340, 1992.
17. Lakier, JB: Smoking and cardiovascular disease. Am J Med 93:8S–12S, 1992.
18. McCulloch, JM, and Kloth, LC: Evaluation of patients with open wounds. In Kloth, LC, McCulloch, JM, and Feedar, JA (eds.): Wound Healing: Alternatives in Management. FA Davis, Philadelphia, 1990, pp 99–118.
19. Browse, NL, and Burnand, KG: The cause of venous ulceration. Lancet 2:243–245, 1982.
20. McCulloch, JM, and Hovde, J: Treatment of wounds due to vascular problems. In Kloth, LC, McCulloch, JM, and Feedar, JA (eds.): Wound Healing: Alternatives in Management. FA Davis, Philadelphia, 1990, pp 177–195.

21. Barnes, RW: Noninvasive tests for chronic venous insufficiency. In Bergan, JJ, and Yao, JST (eds.): Surgery of the Veins. Grune & Stratton, Philadelphia, 1985.

22. Talbot, SR: Use of real time imaging in identifying deep venous obstruction: A preliminary report. Bruit 6:41, 1982.

23. Flanagan, LD, Sullivan, ED, and Cranley, JJ: Venous imaging of the extremities using real time B-mode ultrasound. In Bergan, JJ, and Yao, JST (eds.): Surgery of the Veins. Grune & Stratton, Philadelphia, 1985.

24. Tunis, SR, Bass, EB, Klag, MJ, and Steinberg, EP: Variation in utilization of procedures for treatment of peripheral arterial disease: A look at patient characteristics. Arch Intern Med 153:991–998, 1993.

25. Kloth, LC, McCulloch, JM, and Feedar, JA: Wound Healing: Alternatives in Management. FA Davis, Philadelphia, 1990.

26. McCulloch, J: Peripheral vascular disease. In O'Sullivan, SB, and Schmitz, TJ (eds.): Physical Rehabilitation: Assessment and Treatment, ed 3. FA Davis, Philadelphia, 1994, pp 361–373.

27. Wong, RA: Chronic dermal wounds in older adults. In Guccione, AA (ed.): Geriatric Physical Therapy. Mosby, St. Louis, 1993.

28. Weiss, T, Fujita, Y, Kreimeier, U, and Messmer, K: Effect of intensive walking exercises on skeletal muscle blood flow in intermittent claudication. Angiology 43:63–71, 1992.

29. Burnand, KG, and Layer, G: Graduated elastic stockings. Br Med J 293:224, 1986.

chapter three

The Diabetic Foot

Jeffrey S. Dowling, MHE, PT

OBJECTIVES

At the end of this chapter, all students are expected to:

1   Identify risk factors leading to ulceration.

2   Describe how specific risk factors in clients with diabetes lead to foot dysfunction.

3   Discuss the importance of education in the prevention of ulceration or reulceration in the diabetic population.

4   Describe key elements of the treatment program.

PT students are expected to:

1   Develop an evaluation plan for a client at risk for ulceration or a client with an existing ulceration.

2   Establish short-term and long-term goals for clients with various stages of ulceration.

3   Design a treatment program for clients at various stages of ulceration.

case study

Gladys Greene, a 63-year-old woman with a long history of diabetes, is referred to physical therapy for whirlpool and debridement of a chronic forefoot ulcer (over 4 months in duration) on the plantar aspect of her right foot. She has been coming for outpatient treatment three times a week for the past 3 weeks. She walks into the department bearing full weight on the right lower extremity with no evidence of pain. Her foot is wrapped in a clean dressing with no signs of infection. She wears a house slipper on her right foot and a tennis shoe on her left. Her forefoot ulcer has remained essentially unchanged over the course of nine treatments.

CASE STUDY ACTIVITIES

1 Describe how specific risk factors in clients with diabetes lead to foot dysfunction.

2 Determine which risk factors appear to be contributing to the persistent nature of Ms. Greene's forefoot plantar ulcer.

Pathophysiology and Risk Factors

Ms. Greene's medical records show peripheral vascular disease, although recent studies did not indicate a need for reconstructive surgery. Her persistent forefoot ulcer is apparently related to other factors. Individuals with diabetes have a 15 percent chance of developing ulceration of the foot or ankle during the course of the disease.[1] The foot ulcer, also called mal perforans ulcer, is the most common type of lesion; nearly 90 percent occur in the plantar forefoot region.[2,3] The etiology is unknown, but risk factors include mechanical stress and vascular disease. Approximately 57 to 94 percent of ulcers heal completely, depending on the extent of involvement; however, ulcers place the foot at serious risk of infection and gangrene.[4] Early detection through thorough and frequent inspection of the feet is extremely important. Prompt and aggressive treatment can limit exacerbation.

NEUROPATHY

Neuropathy with some degree of associated sensory, autonomic, and motor involvement is a major cause of diabetic foot lesions.[5] The etiology may be related to the metabolic abnormalities of diabetes. The most common form is distal symmetrical sensorimotor polyneuropathy.

Sensory Neuropathy

Sensory neuropathy is the most important neuropathic risk factor, especially when it involves the small sensory fibers of pain and temperature. The individual develops an insensitive foot more vulnerable to trauma. Sensory neuropathy typically has a stocking-glove type distribution involving the entire extremity distal to the knee. The severity of sensory loss is greatest distally, leaving the toes more susceptible to trauma than the ankle or leg, respectively. With decreased ability to feel pain, the individual may repeatedly traumatize the tissue to the point of ulceration.

Autonomic Neuropathy

Neuropathic involvement of the postganglionic sympathetic fibers to the sweat glands is common. Clinical evaluation reveals dry, noncompliant skin that cracks and splits easily, leaving fissures that are difficult to heal and act as portals for infection. The skin is also susceptible to callus formation under weight bearing areas. A thick callus over a bony prominence increases plantar pressures resulting in greater risk of pressure necrosis and ulceration.[6] Peripheral sympathetic neuropathy (Charcot's foot) may result in demineralization and weakening of the bone and, with repetitive painless trauma, may lead to fracture and deformity.[7] Early signs of bony involvement or fracture are prominent dorsal veins, edema, and increased skin temperature.

Motor Neuropathy

Motor neuropathy frequently contributes to toe deformities. Dysfunction of the intrinsic muscles results in clawing of the lesser toes with hyperextension of the metatarsophalangeal joints and flexion of the proximal interphalangeal joints. Metatarsophalangeal hyperextension depresses the metatarsal heads, increasing the pressure beneath them and contributing to the forces that produce the classic mal perforans ulceration of the forefoot[8] (Fig. 3.1). Flexion contracture at the proximal interphalangeal joint can cause pressure of the toe against the toe box of the shoe, leading to dorsal ulceration. Motor neuropathy can also affect a single major proximal nerve, most often the common peroneal nerve. A significant muscular deficit, such as unilateral foot drop, may occur.

MECHANICAL STRESS

Mechanical stress may be subdivided into parallel (shear) and oblique (perpendicular) components. Bursae and tendon sheaths slide along fascial planes during gait when the foot is firmly planted on the ground creating shear forces.

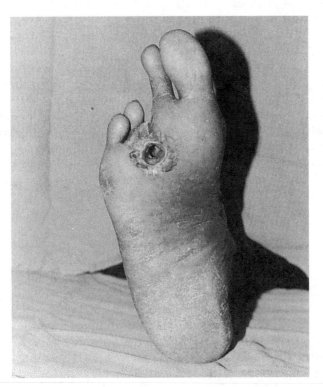

FIGURE 3.1
Mal perforans ulceration on a client with diabetes and severe peripheral neuropathy. Previous amputation of the third toe resulted in increased mechanical stress beneath the metatarsal head, which led to the ulcer formation.

When ulceration occurs and subsequently heals, scarring prevents normal sliding of tissues, leading to creation of new ulcers.

Constant pressure applied perpendicularly for extended periods leads to ischemic necrosis. A tight shoe worn all day applies constant pressure over a bony prominence. Sudden high pressure, such as stepping on a thumbtack or small stone, may also cause injury. Moderate pressure repeated many times without rest, such as during walking, can result in inflammation and may progress to ulceration. Moderate intermittent pressure creates an inflammatory enzymatic autolysis rather than an ischemic necrosis because the blood supply is not continuously blocked.[9]

VASCULAR DISEASE

Chapter 2 outlines the basic concepts of peripheral vascular disease. Vascular disease with resultant circulatory insufficiency does not appear to be a primary cause of foot pathology among individuals with diabetes.[10] It may, however, contribute to tissue damage or compromise wound healing in the presence of the other factors described in this section.

INFECTION

Infection may precede or follow ulceration. Trauma to neuropathic or ischemic tissues can produce an ulcer that may become infected. Alternately, an individual can develop an infection that may cause an ulcer. An interdigital fissure or corn can lead to a large plantar space infection with necrotizing fasciitis. An ulcer will develop when the infection reaches the surface through draining sinuses and necrotic bullae. In either instance, infection frequently leads to formation of microthrombi.[11] When the smaller, distal arteries of the foot are involved, gangrene of the toes is likely. An impaired vascular system also impairs the delivery of systemic antibiotics and oxygen to the involved tissues, making the treatment of infection more difficult.

case study

During a conversation with one of the staff physical therapists (PTs), you are informed that the hospital has a diabetic foot clinic that meets once a month in the orthopedic clinic. You talk with one of the staff orthopedists, who invites you to attend the clinic and gives you several articles on diabetic wound healing, diagnosis, and care of the diabetic foot. You also arrange to have Ms. Greene referred to the clinic by her primary care physician.

CASE STUDY ACTIVITIES

1 Based on the risk factors previously described, list the evaluation procedures you would use to assess a client with diabetes at risk for ulceration.
2 Practice performing any evaluation activities which may be new to you.

Evaluation

HISTORY

The first step in the physical therapy evaluation is a thorough history. The physical therapist (PT) identifies the primary complaint, current associated symptoms, approximate date of onset, and events leading up to foot problem. A history of similar complaints, previous ulcers, and amputations aids in determining the mechanism of injury and the effectiveness or ineffectiveness of past treatment. The PT also determines the individual's understanding of diabetes and its impact on the lower extremities. A person who understands the risk factors related to foot dysfunction is usually more compliant with treatment. The PT and physical therapist assistant (PTA) also need to know the client's level of diabetic control. Although control of diabetes is a specific concern of the physician, it is important that PTs and PTAs understand how it relates to the outcome of treatment. Inadequate control of blood glucose may interfere with normal white blood cell function, making the tissues more susceptible to infection. Glycosylation of structural proteins may occur in an individual with poor control of diabetes.[12] Long-term control of diabetes is possible when the client is taught to monitor blood glucose levels on a routine basis independently.

VISUAL INSPECTION

The PT performs a thorough visual examination of the client's legs, ankles, and feet. With both shoes and socks removed, general overall appearance and any asymmetries are noted. Look for changes in color or texture of the skin, the presence of any deformities, and whether or not any ulcers are present.

NEUROLOGICAL EXAMINATION

Sensory

Vibratory sense is usually the first function lost, followed by decreasing reflex activity, and finally the loss of perception of pain and touch.[11] Pain sensation is easy to assess clinically by use of the Achilles Squeeze Test. The midpoint of the client's Achilles tendon is compressed between the examiner's index finger and thumb with moderate force. This is normally painful, but the individual with significant sensory neuropathy feels only the pressure or nothing at all.[13]

Semmes-Weinstein monofilaments provide an easy and highly predictable method of assessment for touch sensation. The filaments are made of nylon (similar to that used for fishing line) of various diameters set at right angles to an acrylic rod. The filaments are calibrated according to the number of grams of force required to bend the filament. Three filaments (1 gram, 10 grams, and 75 grams) are used in the assessment. The filament is applied to the plantar aspect of the foot with enough force to cause it to buckle. Perception of the 1 gram monofilament is the threshold for normal sensation. The 10 gram monofilament is the threshold for protective sensation, and the person with diabetes who can perceive this pressure is unlikely to sustain major foot trauma.[14] Perception of the 75 gram monofilament or no perception at all indicates an increased risk for ulceration.

Motor

Standard muscle testing is used for static and dynamic strength examinations. Weakness within the foot results in deformities secondary to motor imbalance. Intrinsic weakness predisposes the foot to cavus and claw deformities. Peroneal nerve extrinsic weakness may result in an equinoadductovarus deformity. Tibial nerve extrinsic weakness may result in a calcaneoabductovalgus deformity. A gross evaluation beginning by having the client walk on the heels and then the toes is followed by a more detailed muscle examination.

VASCULAR EXAMINATION

The femoral, popliteal, posterior tibial, and dorsalis pedis pulses are palpated; pulses are graded as 2+ = normal, 1+ = diminished, and 0 = absent. A significantly decreased or absent pulse is often associated with atherosclerotic disease.

Capillary refilling time from the arteriolar blood supply is assessed by blanching the toe pulps with pressure by the fingertips. The time taken for the return of normal color is counted in seconds. The normal range of refill is up to 3 seconds; longer periods of time are considered delays.

The most readily available and productive information about vascular integrity can be obtained through the use of a Doppler device. Doppler units can measure the vascular status by determining the ratio of systolic blood pressure in the foot to that in the arm.[14] These units are small and portable, and provide quick and objective measurements concerning the vascular supply (see Chap. 2).

MUSCULOSKELETAL EXAMINATION

A thorough and firm palpation of the foot is done. Palpation may reveal a plantar fascial inflammation in the presence of ulceration and possible infection; it is also an indicator of deep plantar space involvement. Palpation can help identify the amount of motion available in a particular joint. Limited range of motion may result from neuroarthropathy or soft tissue scarring from previous inflammation and scarring.

ASSESSMENT OF EXISTING AND POTENTIAL ULCERS

An injury to the diabetic foot can be classified as either a potential ulceration (preulceration) or a complete ulceration. A preulceration is any undesirable change to the intact skin that, if left untreated, will be likely to progress to a complete ulceration.[10] Preulcers may exhibit one or a combination of the following changes: (1) increased temperature in a localized region in comparison to the contralateral foot and in the absence of significant physical activity before assessment; (2) maceration of the intraepidermal layer that creates a boggy texture in the skin similar to that seen with an intact blister; with or without (3) a hematoma or a callus with an underlying hematoma.

If the individual presents with a complete ulcer, the dimensions of the wound are measured and the lesion is graded according to its depth and the tissue involved. Wound tracings on sterile acetate film may be more useful than

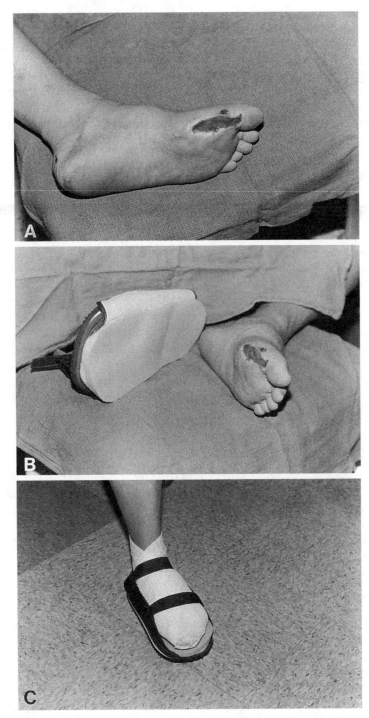

F I G U R E   3 . 2

(*A*) Mal perforans ulceration beneath the first metatarsal head. (*B*) Plastizote liner contoured and bonded to a cast shoe to provide a pressure relief area beneath the first metatarsal head. (*C*) The client is encouraged to bear weight on the posterior aspect of the shoe further to decrease stress to the forefoot region.

T A B L E   3 . 1   **ULCER CLASSIFICATION SYSTEM**

0	No skin lesions
1	Dense callus lesions but no preulcer or ulcer
2	Preulcerative changes
3	Partial thickness (superficial) ulcer
4	Full thickness (deep) ulcer but no involvement of tendon, bone, ligament, or joint
5	Full thickness (deep) ulcer with involvement of tendon, bone, ligament, or joint
6	Localized infection (abscess or osteomyelitis) in foot
7	Proximal spread of infection (ascending cellulitis or lymphadenopathy)
8	Gangrene of forefoot only
9	Gangrene of most of foot

Source: Adapted from Sims, DS, Cavanagh, PR, and Ulbrecht, JS: Risk factors in the diabetic foot: Recognition and management. Reprinted from Phys Ther 68(12):1887, 1988 with permission of the American Physical Therapy Association.

diameter measurements if the borders are irregular (Fig. 3.2). Serial drawings may be compared visually or digitized electronically to obtain area measurements. Photographs provide another means of documenting wound location and size. A cardinal sign of a deep ulcer that has penetrated a joint capsule is the production of a clear fluid with bubbles.

ULCER CLASSIFICATION

The most widely accepted classification system for diabetic foot ulcers and lesions is based on the depth of penetration and extent of tissue necrosis. Six categories or grades range from 0 to 5. A grade of 0 is used to describe intact normal skin, grades 1 through 4 indicate progressive stages of tissue destruction, and grade 5 indicates extensive gangrene or necrosis and a need for amputation.[15]

An alternate ulcer classification system emphasizes the importance of early identification of foot problems in the prevention of plantar ulcers and the nonsurgical treatment of ulcerations as contrasted to the Wagner system, which emphasizes surgical treatment (Table 3.1).[10]

case study

Figure 3.3 is the PT evaluation for Ms. Gladys Greene.

CASE STUDY ACTIVITIES

PT Students

1   Based on the findings, decide on your short term and long term goals for Ms. Greene.

2   Using the results of the evaluation, develop a treatment plan for Ms. Greene.

SUBJECTIVE EXAM:

Chief complaint:	Non-healing plantar ulcer right foot
Mechanism of injury:	No known direct trauma, probable repetitive low level stress
Associated symptoms:	Moderate amount serosanguinous drainage
Onset:	Approximately 4 months ago
Previous ulcerations/amputation:	Amputation of gangrenous 2nd digit right foot (approx. 2 years ago)
Diabetic education:	None related to foot care
Diabetic control:	Good

OBJECTIVE EXAM:

Visual:	Right foot moderately edematous with slightly increased temperature; flattened arch (rocker bottom appearance); hammer toe deformities of lesser toes; 2nd digit absent with well healed scar in web space; plantar ulceration 1st metatarsal head
Sensory:	Lacks protective sensation plantar aspect right foot
Motor:	No palpable contraction of the intrinsic muscles of right foot; weak anterior crural musculature of right leg
Vascular:	1+ pulses posterior tibial and dorsalis pedis arteries on right; decreased but adequate bloodflow per Doppler study (approx> 1 yr ago)
MusSkel:	Contracture lesser toes 3, 4, 5, limited dorsiflexion 1st MP joint; minimal forefoot and subtalar joint motion; ankle DF=0; ankle PF=35
Wound:	Grade 5 ulceration (Table 3.1); 2.5 cm diameter; exposed flexor tendon; no joint space involvement; no signs of infection

* For the purpose of this chapter, the information regarding the examination of the left foot was not included. An actual examination must include information regarding both extremities.

FIGURE 3.3
Physical therapy evaluation for Gladys Greene.

PTA Students

1 What do you think the goals of treatment will be?
2 What parts of the treatment program would you expect to have delegated to you?

Medical Management

REVASCULARIZATION

Initially, plantar ulcers may be treated medically and nonsurgically; however, if conservative approaches fail, revascularization surgery may be required.

SURGICAL CORRECTION OF DEFORMITY

Prophylactic surgical correction, such as toenail modification and removal, hammer and claw toe repairs, bunionectomies, metatarsal head resections, metatarsal osteotomies, and resections of bony prominences are performed to reduce pressure areas. Shoe modification and orthotic devices are alternatives to surgery if the deformities are limited or surgical risks too high.[5]

TREATMENT OF INFECTION

Infection is the most common reason for amputation and is a serious threat to the limb and the life of the individual.[5] Superficial infections are usually treated with local wound care. Deep infections require surgical incision and drainage as well as the use of systemic antibiotics. An abscess is the most common type of infection in the diabetic foot.[16] The abscess must be completely opened and the infected tissue removed to increase the effectiveness of treatment. The client must also remain nonweight bearing during healing to prevent spread of infection to other regions of the foot.[17] Broad spectrum antibiotics or a combination of two or more antibiotics can be used initially until the specific organism is identified and treated with the most appropriate drug.

NAIL AND SKIN CARE

Toenail abnormalities, particularly thickening of the nails (onychogryphosis) secondary to fungal infections, are common.[18] The thickened nail may lead to necrosis, subungual hemorrhage, and ulceration at the nailbed caused by pressure from improperly fitted shoes. Nails that are allowed to grow too long may curve into a neighboring toe and cause a laceration or ulceration.[19] The client also risks injury when performing "bathroom surgery" to remove an ingrown toenail or when trimming the nails with a sharp instrument, such as a pointed nail file or razor blade.

Autonomic neuropathy can cause the skin of the feet to be excessively dry, leading to cracks and fissures. Parts of the foot exposed to mechanical stress may develop excessively thick calluses, which also increase the risk of pressure necrosis. Any injury can lead to infection and gangrene. The client or a family member needs to learn proper nail and skin care. Professional intervention may be required, especially in the management of hypertrophic nails and thick calluses.

Physical Therapy Management

WOUND CARE

The wound should be debrided, cleaned, and covered with dressings using sterile technique and universal precautions. A heavy callus typically forms around the border of the ulcer and should be trimmed to promote epithelial growth. A topical antiseptic effective against bacteria found on the wound is also beneficial. No specific topical agent has been found to have any major contribution to the healing rate of neuropathic ulcers.[20]

DECREASING PRESSURE DURING HEALING

Reducing weight bearing stresses on the foot by decreasing weight bearing is critical to healing an ulcer. The many ways of reducing weight bearing include bed rest, special shoes and sandals, and total contact casts.

Bed Rest

Bed rest is the simplest method to reduce weight bearing but it is the least practical or effective because strict compliance is rare. In the absence of normal pain perception, the individual may still continue to walk short distances in the house, bearing weight on the unprotected and ulcerated foot. Because wound healing may take many months, prolonged periods of bed rest have adverse effects on the person's general health, making this treatment option the least favorable.[13]

Healing Sandals and Shoes

The use of special sandals or shoes is another method of reducing plantar pressure. These sandals and shoes are available commercially and are inexpensive, lightweight, and easily modified. Most are constructed of several layers of heat-moldable polyethylene foam with Plastizote (United Foam Plastics, Georgetown, MA) for insole construction. Plastizote is a nontoxic, closed cell foam that does not absorb body fluids and can be washed with soap and water without damage. It has a low specific heat and can be molded directly over the foot while the Plastizote is still warm. Portions of the polyethylene insole may also be cut out directly beneath the lesion to create areas of greatest pressure relief (Fig. 3.4). The foam will "bottom out" or flatten under areas of high pressure over several months. The material must be replaced when it no longer provides relief from pressure. Compliance may also be a problem because the individual may choose to walk on the ulcerated foot rather than wear the shoe.

Total Contact Casts

The use of total contact plaster casts is well documented and remains the standard by which all other methods of ulcer treatment are measured.[21] The major

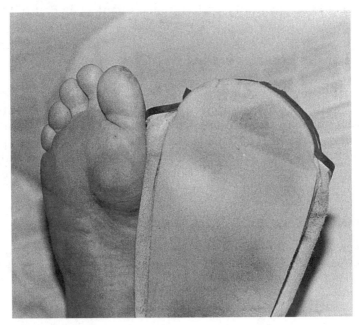

FIGURE 3.4
Plastizote liner after approximately 1 month's wear. Note the areas where the liner has *bottomed out* beneath the first metatarsal head and lateral border of the foot.

difference between traditional fracture casting and total contact casting is the amount of padding applied beneath the casting material. In fracture casting, thick, bulky padding is placed between the skin and the plaster. The total contact casting uses a single layer of cotton stockinette between the skin and plaster. The wound is first assessed, then dressed with a single gauze pad. The leg and foot are covered with stockinette; the bony prominences are padded with orthopedic felt. The innermost layers of plaster are carefully molded over the foot and leg to obtain optimal contact and the outer layers are applied primarily for added stability. The distal end is closed to prevent debris from entering the cast, which could traumatize the insensitive foot. The initial cast is left on no longer than 1 week and must be changed sooner if excessive loosening occurs. The ulcer is reevaluated, and then the cast is reapplied. Subsequent casts are replaced approximately every 2 weeks. At each cast removal or reapplication, the ulcer is reevaluated. Once the ulcer has healed, the foot should be placed in appropriate therapeutic footwear to prevent reulceration.

The effectiveness of the cast is partly related to its ability to protect the ulcer from direct trauma; to reduce edema, which may inhibit blood flow to the healing tissues; and to immobilize the joints and soft tissue surrounding the ulceration. Compliance is not an issue because the device cannot be removed without a cast cutter. The greatest benefit comes from the cast's ability to reduce the concentration of stress at the site of the ulcer by dissipating the forces across the plantar surface of the foot while maintaining ambulation. Reductions of as much as 75 to 84 percent of peak pressure over the first and third metatarsal heads have been reported in individuals walking in total contact casts compared to those wearing normal shoes.[22] The average length of time for complete wound closure using this method of treatment is from 5 to 6 weeks.[23–25]

CASE STUDY ACTIVITY

Assume that your treatment was successful and wound closure was obtained. Develop a plan for Ms. Greene that will reduce her risk of future ulceration or reulceration. Be sure to address areas of specific footwear and education.

General Management

PREVENTION

Many factors may contribute to ulcer development; however, the degree to which each factor contributes to tissue destruction is unclear. Minimizing the known factors reduces the risk of ulceration or reulceration and improves the healing potential.

RISK CLASSIFICATION

Prevention begins with a comprehensive evaluation. The client may then be categorized according to the degree of risk for injury or reinjury. Risk classification is based on the individual's level of protective sensation, the degree of deformity that may contribute in increased plantar pressures, and the history

T A B L E   3 . 2   **RISK AND MANAGEMENT CATEGORIES**

Risk	Management
Category 0	
Protective sensation	Foot clinic once per year
May have a foot deformity	Client education to include proper selection of shoe
Has a disease that could lead to insensitivity	style
Category 1	
Protective sensation absent	Foot clinic every 6 months
No history of plantar ulceration	Review client's current footwear
No foot deformity	Add soft insoles (Spenco[1], nylon covered PPT[2])
Category 2	
Protective sensation absent	Foot clinic every 3–4 months
No history of plantar ulcer	Custom molded orthotic devices are usually indicated
Foot deformity present	Prescription shoes are often required
Category 3	
Protective sensation absent	Foot clinic every 1–2 months
There is a history of foot ulceration with vascular laboratory findings; indicate significant vascular disease	Custom orthotic devices are necessary Prescription shoes are often required

Source: Levin, ME, O'Neal, LW, and Bowker, JH (eds): The Diabetic Foot. ed 5, C.V. Mosby, St. Louis,
    1993, p 534, with permission.
[1]Spenco Medical Corporation, Waco, TX.
[2]Professional Protective Technology, Deer Park, NY.

of previous injury that may increase the foot's vulnerability to future injury (Table 3.2).

RISK MANAGEMENT

Management is based on the level of risk. Individuals at a higher risk of ulceration need to have their feet professionally examined more frequently than those in a lower risk category. Individuals at a higher risk may need specific insoles, custom molded devices, or prescription footwear. Individuals at lower risk may require only education on proper footwear selection (see Table 3.2).

EDUCATION

Self-Inspection

The client should be taught to perform twice daily foot inspection, at the beginning and end of the day. More frequent inspection may be required during periods of abnormally high activity and while breaking in new shoes. The client should inspect each foot in a well lit place. If the individual has difficulty placing the foot in a position that allows for a thorough visual inspection, a wall mounted or handheld mirror may be helpful. If the individual has impaired vision, inspection should be performed by a friend or family member. Above all, whoever inspects the foot must be able to recognize the warning signs and know how to respond to them most appropriately.

Foot Care

In addition to self-inspection, the client should be instructed in daily foot care.[26] Individuals with diabetes should wash their feet thoroughly using warm, soapy water and a soft washcloth. The feet should be dried completely, especially between the toes, to prevent maceration of the skin. Any water based lotion may be applied to keep the skin soft and pliable. Lotion should not be applied between the toes. Nails are trimmed straight across with clippers, avoiding rounding of the corners; it is safest to file the nails regularly with an emery board. Thickened calluses may be safely reduced with a foot file or pumice stone. Care of thick nails or calluses requires the assistance of a trained family member or professional.

Footwear Considerations

Proper footwear is one of the most important considerations in the prevention of ulceration or reulceration in the case of a newly healed ulcer. Shoes and orthotic devices should be selected based on the level of risk for injury.[10] Those at lowest risk should select leather shoes because this material adapts to the contours of the foot over time better than synthetic materials. The heel and midfoot section should fit securely on the foot to prevent slippage; the toe box should be sufficiently high and wide and at least 1 centimeter (about ⅜ inch) longer than the longest toe to prevent crowding and pressure on the toes. Shoes manufactured with an extra deep toe box should be selected when deformities,

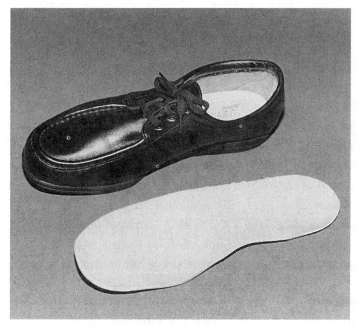

FIGURE 3.5
Extra depth shoe with removable foam liner. Note how the liner has begun to be contoured to the shape of the foot after less than 1 week of wear.

such as claw toes, are present. Extra depth is extremely important if additional insole material is to be added to the shoe.

Individuals with impaired sensation and deformity require custom molded inserts made from soft thermoplastic materials (Fig. 3.5). Individuals with severe deformity require a custom molded shoe or boot. Custom molded footwear is relatively expensive but may be necessary to adequately accommodate the deformity. However, cost is relative when considering the cost of wound care, amputation, prosthetics, and rehabilitation following amputation.

Cotton and wool socks provide the best padding between the foot and shoe. The socks should be clean, in good condition without holes, and without wrinkles and folds. White socks are preferable to colored because dyes may cause irritation. The shoes should be inspected inside for foreign objects before each wearing. They should be in good repair and free from tacks or nails that can pierce the insole and project into the foot. New shoes should be worn no more than 2 hours per day for the first week. Wear may be extended an additional 2 hours each succeeding week.

SUMMARY

Ulceration of the diabetic foot is a common problem that can ultimately result in amputation; however, most ulcers heal if managed properly. Professionals who care for individuals with diabetes must be able to identify the risk factors contributing to delayed healing and to know methods to reduce these factors. Above all, prevention is the ultimate goal, with emphasis placed on education. Long-term security for the diabetic foot is maximized when individuals accept responsibility for the routine inspection and care of their own feet.

GLOSSARY

Autolysis	Self dissolution of tissue, usually by an enzyme within the body.
Bulla	A large fluid filled blister.
Callus	A hypertrophied or thickened area of the skin.
Debridement	Removal of dead or damaged tissue from a wound.
Fissure	A cracklike opening in the skin.
Gangrene or necrosis	Death of tissue, usually caused by lack of circulation.
Glycosylation	Excess sugars in the cells.
Hematoma	A swelling or mass of blood.
Ischemia	Lack of blood to an area or part.
Neuroarthropathy	Joint disease combined with central nervous system disorder.
Neuropathy	A disease of the nervous system.
Sinus	A canal or passage.
Subungual	Located beneath a fingernail or toenail.

REFERENCES

1. Palumbo, PJ, and Melton, LJ: Peripheral vascular disease and diabetes. In Harris, MI, and Hamman, RF (eds.): Diabetes in America. National Institutes of Health, Bethesda, NIH pub. no. 85-1468, 1985, p XV, 1–21.
2. Birke, JA, and Sims, DS: Plantar sensory threshold in the ulcerative foot. Lepr Rev 57:261, 1986.
3. Sabato, S, Yosipovitch, Z, Simkin, A, and Sheskin, J: Plantar trophic ulcers in patients with leprosy: A correlative study of sensation, pressure and mobility. Int Orthop 6:203, 1982.
4. Reiber, G: Epidemiology of the diabetic foot. In Levin, ME, O'Neal, LW, and Bowker, JH (eds.): The Diabetic Foot, ed 5. Mosby, St. Louis, 1993, pp 1–15.
5. Brodsky, JW: The diabetic foot. In Mann, RA, and Coughlin, MJ (eds.): Surgery of the Foot and Ankle, ed 6. Mosby-Year Book, St. Louis, 1993, pp 877–958.
6. Bell, DS: Lower limb problems in diabetics: What are the causes?: What are the remedies? Post Grad Med 89:237, 1991.
7. Levin, ME: Medical management of the diabetic foot. In Kerstein, MD (ed.): Diabetes and Vascular Disease. JB Lippincott, Philadelphia, 1990, pp 193–213.
8. Hamptom, G, and Birke, J: Treatment of wounds caused by pressure and insensitivity. In Kloth, LC, McCulloch, JM, and Feedar, JA (eds.): Wound Healing: Alternatives in Management. FA Davis, Philadelphia, 1990, pp 196–220.
9. Brand, PW: The diabetic foot. In Ellenberg, M, and Rifkin, H (eds.): Diabetes Mellitus: Theory and Practice, ed 3. Medical Examination Publishing Co. Inc., New Hyde Park, NY, 1983, pp 829–849.
10. Sims, DS, Cavanagh, PR, and Ulbrecht, JS: Risk factors in the diabetic foot: Recognition and management. Phys Ther 68:1887, 1988.
11. Levin, ME: Diabetic foot lesions. In Young, JR, Graor, RA, Olin, JW, and Bartholomew, JR (eds.): Peripheral Vascular Disease. Mosby-Year Book, St. Louis, 1991, pp 669–711.
12. Delbridge, L, et al: Nonenzymatic glycosylation of keratin from the stratum corneum of the diabetic foot. Br J Dermatol 112:547, 1985.
13. Levine, MI: Personal communication, December 1993.
14. Birke, JA, and Sims, DS: Plantar sensory threshold in the ulcerative foot. Lepr Rev 57:261, 1986.
15. Wagner, FW: The dysvascular foot: A system for diagnosis and treatment. Foot Ankle 2:64, 1981.
16. Schwartz, N: The diabetic foot. In Donatelli, R (ed.): The Biomechanics of the Foot and Ankle. FA Davis, Philadelphia, 1990, pp 178–189.
17. Brand, PW: Management of the insensitive limb. Phys Ther 59:8, 1979.
18. Little, JR, Kobayashi, GS, and Bailey, TC: Infection of the diabetic foot.. In Levin, ME, O'Neal, LW, and Bowker, JH (eds.): The Diabetic Foot, ed 5. Mosby, St. Louis, 1993, pp 181–198.
19. O'Neal, LW: Surgical pathology of the foot and clinicopathology correlations. In Levin, ME, O'Neal, LW, and Bowker, JH (eds.): The Diabetic Foot, ed 5. Mosby, St. Louis, 1993, pp 457–491.
20. Birke JA, Novick, A, Graham, SL, Coleman, WC, and Brasseaux, DM: Methods of treating plantar ulcers. Phys Ther 71:116, 1991.
21. Birke, JA, Sims, DA, and Buford, WL: Walking casts: Effect of plantar foot pressures. J Rehabil Res Dev 22:18, 1985.
22. Laing, PW, Cogley, DI, and Klenerman, L: Neuropathic foot ulceration treated by total contact casts. J Bone Joint Surg 74B:133, 1992.
23. Sinacore, DR, Mueller, MJ, Diamond, JE, Blair, VP, Drury, D, and Rose, SJ: Diabetic plantar ulcers treated by total contact casting. Phys Ther 67:1543, 1987.
24. Walker, SC, Helm, PA, and Pullium, G: Total contact casting and chronic diabetic neuropathic foot ulcerations: Healing rates by wound location. Arch Phys Med Rehabil 68:217, 1987.
25. Birke, JA, Koziatek, E, and Coleman, WC: Healing rates in diabetic and non-diabetic plantar ulcers. Unpublished study, 1988.
26. Eramo-Melkus, GD: Education and counseling for diabetes self-care. In Gambert, SR: Diabetes Mellitus in the Elderly. Raven Press, New York, 1990, pp 207–225.

chapter four

Lower Extremity Amputation Surgery

OBJECTIVES

At the end of this chapter, all students are expected to:

1 Describe the process of amputation surgery in relation to residual limb characteristics and function.

2 Describe the functional results of amputation surgery.

case studies

The following clients have been referred to physical therapy for evaluation and treatment:

Diana Magnolia: she underwent a left transtibial amputation yesterday secondary to diabetic gangrene.

Benny Pearl: a right transfemoral amputation was done yesterday secondary to chronic atherosclerosis obliterans.

Ha Lee Davis: an 18-year-old man underwent traumatic transtibial amputation secondary to a motorcycle accident 2 days ago.

Betty Childs: a 12-year-old girl underwent a transfemoral amputation yesterday secondary to IIB osteogenic sarcoma of the proximal right tibia.

CASE STUDY ACTIVITIES

All Students:

For each client, describe what the surgeon will do with the bone, blood vessels, nerves, muscle tissue, and skin.

Physical Therapy Students:

Identify what you need to know about amputation surgery to plan an evaluation and treatment program.

Physical Therapist Assistant Students:

Identify what you need to know about amputation surgery to carry out a treatment program.

Most lower extremity amputations are performed secondary to peripheral vascular disease (> 90%). Usually, amputation is preceded by attempts at limb salvage through revascularization procedures (see Chap. 2). The level of amputation is determined by the healing potential of the residual limb and the general health of the client. Successful healing does not require patency of major vessels but does need patency of small vessels in the skin.[1-3] Surgeons use various methods to determine the lowest possible level that is likely to heal, such as skin temperature, palpable pulses, and blood flow measures.[3] Amputations for peripheral vascular disease are usually performed through the foot, through the tibia (transtibial), or through the femur (transfemoral). Disarticulations are not usually performed for limb ischemia because the lower vascularization in the joints mitigates against successful healing. Many studies show poor success rates for ankle disarticulation in the presence of severe limb ischemia.[1]

Level selection for traumatic amputations or for major tumors is determined by the nature of the injury and the viability of tissues. The incidence of amputation for tumors has decreased with the advent of improved detection and chemotherapeutic management of tumors. Whenever possible, the tumor is excised and the bone replaced with a metal implant or an allograft, eliminating the need for amputation. Rates for 5 year survival have been about the same for individuals undergoing amputation and those having segmental excisions. Amputations are generally performed on individuals with large tumors who do not respond well to preoperative chemotherapy.[3]

General Principles

Several principles of amputation surgery apply to all levels of amputation. Because most amputations are made necessary by vascular disease, they are performed by vascular surgeons who are not required to study prosthetic rehabilitation. Orthopedic surgeons, who perform most of the nonvascular amputations, must take courses in prosthetic rehabilitation.

Generally, surgeons want to save as much length as possible while providing a residual limb that is able to tolerate the stresses of the prosthesis and of mobility activities. Sometimes, compromises are necessary between keeping bone length and avoiding scars and other deformities that may interfere with prosthetic fitting (Fig. 4.1).

Major nerves are pulled down firmly, resected sharply, and allowed to retract into the soft tissue. When severed, all peripheral nerves put out new tendrils that form into small neoplasms of nerve ends (neuromas). Size and location of the neuroma are critical. If small and imbedded in soft tissue, it is usually not a problem. If the neuroma is large or superficial, or becomes squeezed against a bone, it can cause pain. Resecting the nerves under tension usually prevents such problems.

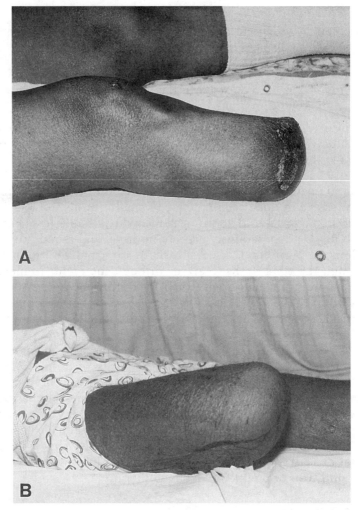

FIGURE 4.1
(*A*) Residual limb after transtibial amputation. (*B*) Residual limb after transfemoral amputation.

Muscle and soft tissue are differentially handled depending on the level of amputation. When a muscle is severed, it loses its distal attachment and, if left loose, will retract, atrophy, and scar against adjacent structures. Without attachment at both ends, a muscle is unable to function. Muscles can be managed in two ways. The term **myoplasty** refers to the attachment of anterior and posterior compartment muscles to each other over the end of the bone. Myoplasty is usually performed in through the bone amputations and incorporated with myofascial closure to provide muscle stability, making sure the muscles do not slide over the end of the bone. The term **myodesis** refers to the anchoring of muscles to bone. Myodesis is performed more rarely because it requires a longer surgical procedure and causes more trauma to the bone itself. In both instances, muscles are stabilized under a little tension to provide a well shaped residual limb.

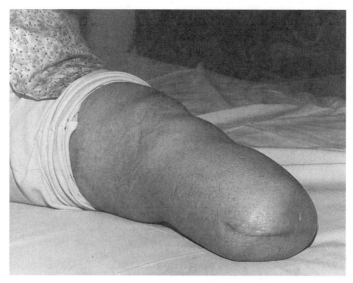

FIGURE 4.2
Residual limb from a transtibial amputation with suture of equal length flaps. (With permission from May, BJ: Assessment and treatment of individuals following lower extremity amputation. In O'Sullivan, SB, and Schmitz, TJ (eds): Physical Rehabilitation: Assessment and Treatment, ed 3. FA Davis, Philadelphia, 1994, p 377.)

Skin flaps are usually as broad as the distal end of the limb and are shaped to allow the corners to retract smoothly. Anterior and posterior skin flaps place the scar in a medio/lateral direction at the end of the residual limb (Fig. 4.2). Anterior and posterior skin flaps of equal length are generally used except for transtibial amputations for dysvascular problems. Types of postsurgical dressings vary and are discussed in more detail in Chapter 5. A drain is often inserted just under the incision to allow evacuation of excess fluid. The drain is usually removed 1 or 2 days after surgery.

Transtibial (Below Knee) Amputation

The transtibial amputation is the most common level of extremity amputation necessitated by peripheral vascular disease. Prosthetic rehabilitation is more successful and postoperative mortality lower with transtibial compared with transfemoral amputations. Several studies confirm a mortality rate of 9.5 percent following transtibial amputation against 29.5 percent following transfemoral amputation.[4,5] Traditionally, transfemoral amputations were preferred in the presence of peripheral vascular disease because it was thought that the larger vessels enhanced healing. However, studies performed in the 1960s indicated that primary healing could be obtained consistently at transtibial levels.[4,5] Bowker et al. pooled the results of several studies and reported a primary healing rate of 70 percent and secondary healing rate of 16 percent for transtibial amputations.[4] A British study of 713 clients who had amputations at transtibial levels because of ischemia indicated that healing was enhanced by previous attempts at revascularization that increased oxygen to the tissues.[6]

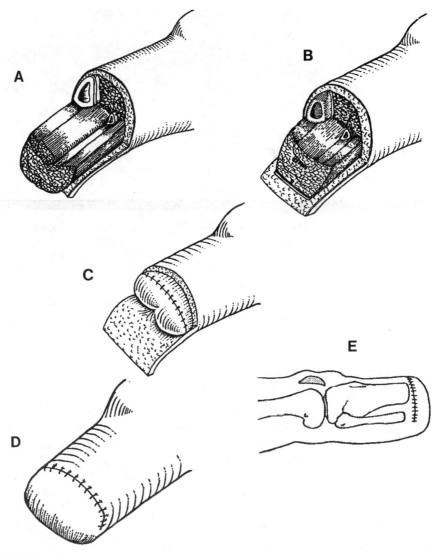

FIGURE 4.3
Transtibial amputation with long posterior skin flap. (*A*) The surgeon leaves a long posterior skin flap. (*B*) The surgeon bevels and contours the flap for a smooth distal end. (*C*) After myoplasty, the soft tissues are approximated. (*D*) The final suture is over the anterior part of the residual limb. (*E*) The relationship of the tibia and fibula.

The specific level of transtibial amputation is determined by several factors. In amputations following trauma, the amount of remaining viable tissue determines the level. In the presence of dysvascular disease with infection, the level is determined by the infection free tissue and the vascular condition of skin flaps and soft tissue. Patency of major vessels is not necessarily a criterion for selecting a level because amputations consistently heal primarily in the absence of circulation through the major vessels if there is bleeding through the skin flaps. The desirable length for a transtibial amputation is a matter of controversy. Some surgeons advocate leaving as much bone length as possible, believing that the longer lever arm decreases the energy required for effective ambulation.[7-10] Others state that individuals with very long residual limbs develop distal skin problems because of the lack of subcutaneous padding.[11] Some surgeons suggest that about 15 centimeters is optimal length.[12] The tibial tubercle is the shortest level of transtibial amputation compatible with knee function.

Today, most surgeons use a long posterior skin flap when performing an amputation for vascular insufficiency (Fig. 4.3). The skin over the posterior leg has a better blood supply than the skin over the anterior leg. The anterior skin flap is cut at approximately the level of anticipated section of the tibia and the posterior flap is 13 to 15 centimeters longer to ensure adequate coverage without undue tension. Dissection is carried down through the deep fascia to the bone. The muscles are divided, blood vessels ligated and divided, and the nerves severed high with a sharp scalpel and then allowed to retract into the soft tissue. The tibia and fibula are sectioned, with the fibula usually cut about 1 centimeter shorter than the tibia for proper shaping of the distal residual limb. Cutting the fibula much shorter than the tibia results in a sharp distal end that may be painful when the client is wearing a prosthesis. Leaving the fibula the same length as the tibia may produce a square end that is more difficult to fit. When amputation is performed at the tibial tubercle level, the fibula is removed because the biceps tendon tends to deviate the small bony remnant that is no longer anchored by soft tissue. The tibia must be beveled anteriorly at a 45° to 60° angle to allow for distribution of distal end pressure over as wide an area as possible and to prevent osteophyte formation. Care is taken to avoid any rough bony areas. Myoplasty is usually preferred over myodesis in the presence of vascular disease; the posterior muscle mass is beveled to allow the flap to come forward and sutured anteriorly to the deep fascia of the anterolateral muscle group and to the periosteum that is reflected over the anterior aspect of the tibia. The skin is brought forward and sutured. The resulting anterior scar usually presents no problem in limb fitting (Fig. 4.4).

When amputation is performed for other than vascular reasons, flaps of equal length are used and the resultant scar is at the distal end of the limb. Equal length flaps are often referred to as a "fish mouth incision" because the shape of the flaps before they are sutured resembles that of a fish's mouth. Equal length flaps allow for less redundant tissue at the end of the residual limb and properly shaped flaps reduce the *dog ears* or excess tissue at the medial and lateral corners that may result from long posterior flaps.

Although the physical therapist (PT) and physical therapist assistant (PTA) have little input into the surgical technique, they need to understand what the surgeon has done to provide for effective postsurgical handling.

Transfemoral (Above Knee) Amputation

Historically, the transfemoral level was the most common for amputation in individuals with impaired circulation and gangrene of the foot and toes. Improved circulation above the knee increased the chances of primary healing. As indicated in Chapter 8, however, ambulation with a transfemoral prosthesis requires considerable energy; many individuals with vascular disease never do become functional walkers. In the past 30 years, the trend has changed as re-

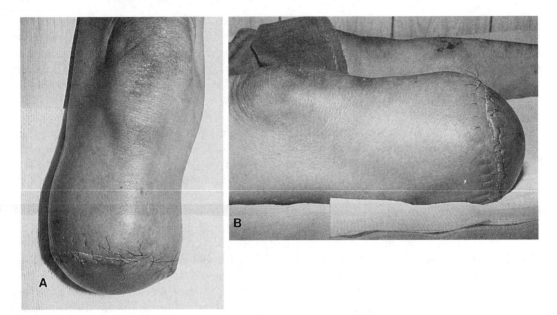

FIGURE 4.4
(A and B) Residual limb from a transtibial amputation, showing the anterior suture from a long posterior flap. (With permission from May, BJ: Assessment and treatment of individuals following lower extremity amputation. In O'Sullivan, SB, and Schmitz, TJ (eds): Physical Rehabilitation: Assessment and Treatment, ed 3. FA Davis, Philadelphia, 1994, p 377.)

search indicated that amputations at the transtibial level heal successfully. Today, more transtibial than transfemoral amputations are performed because of vascular problems. The transfemoral level is still indicated if gangrene has extended to the knee or the client's circulatory status precludes healing at the transtibial level. Trauma is the other major cause of transfemoral amputation, and some procedures are also done for osteomyelitis or tumors. Survival and functional prosthetic rehabilitation rates are lower among individuals who have had transfemoral amputations. Individuals undergoing this procedure are generally sicker and have less energy reserves than individuals with amputations at transtibial levels.

Equal length anterior and posterior flaps are generally used. The thigh muscles and periosteum are divided cleanly to the bone at a length just beyond the most distal part of the skin flaps. For a myoplasty, the thigh muscles are divided into four groups and elevated from the femur back to the level of proposed bone section. The blood vessels are transected just proximal to the level of bone section. The nerves are cut at a level to ensure their being well covered by muscle and remote from the incision. If a neuroma becomes attached to the distal scar, it may displace during walking, causing pain. The femur is divided and the sharp peripheral edges rounded with a rasp. Usually, the adductor magnus tendon is brought around the distal femur and sutured to the lateral distal aspect through small drill holes. The femur is held in adduction to ensure maximum tension on the muscle. The quadriceps and hamstrings are then either anchored to each other over the end of the bone or the quadriceps is attached directly to the femur through small drill holes with the hamstrings attached to the posterior part of the adductor magnus. Regardless of technique, the surgeon attempts to provide muscle stabilization to improve residual limb function. Some surgeons believe that myodesis is necessary to ensure adequate muscle stabilization, whereas others suggest that myoplasty is adequate.[13–16] Some function is lost as muscles are shortened and the femur is no longer held in its normal adducted position by the tibia and fibula. (The resulting effect on gait is discussed in Chap. 8.) The muscles are trimmed before suturing and the skin flaps closed without undue tension with the femur in a neutral position (see Fig. 4.1b). The residual limb may be placed in a rigid dressing or in a compressive wrap.

Amputations at Other Levels

AMPUTATIONS THROUGH THE FOOT

Toe or Ray Amputation (Transphalangeal, Digital Amputation)

Toe amputations are generally indicated for localized demarcated gangrene of the distal end of the toe. A single toe can be amputated through the phalanx or disarticulated, at the base of the proximal phalanx. PTs and PTAs are rarely involved with primary toe amputations, although clients with other levels of amputation may have lost one or more toes on the other side.

On occasion, an entire ray (toe plus metatarsal) must be removed. The metatarsal ray resection is indicated in some cases of congenital anomalies, gangrene secondary to frostbite, neoplasms, severe chronic infections of a single metatarsal, or a deep subaponeurotic foot abscess.

Transmetatarsal Amputation

Transmetatarsal amputation (Fig. 4.5) is removal of the toes and distal ends of the metatarsals. It is a very functional amputation for problems with toes but requires a properly fitting prosthetic replacement. Foot balance is maintained because the residual limb is symmetrical in shape and major muscle attachments are preserved. Transmetatarsal amputations heal relatively slowly because of the limited blood supply on the dorsum, where the incision is located. Once healed, the foot has been shown to survive without the need for further surgery in about 71 percent of cases.[17] The incision is vulnerable to abrasion during the latter part of stance phase.

DISARTICULATION

Both advantages and disadvantages to disarticulations over through bone amputations exist. Disarticulation provides for a residual limb with an intact bone, lowers the chances of osteomyelitis, and in children, maintains intact growth plates. The complete bone length of the disarticulated limb provides for a better lever arm and more prosthetic control, particularly for ankle and knee disarticulations. The disadvantages are decreased cosmesis of the prosthetic replacement and fewer available components to fit the smaller joint space.

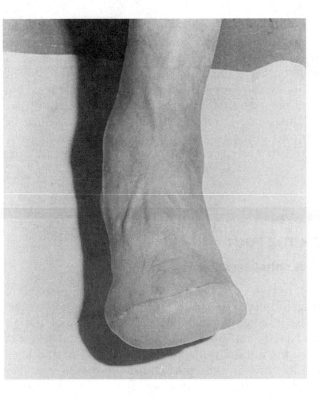

FIGURE 4.5
(*A*) Residual limb after a transmetatarsal amputation.

Ankle Disarticulations

The most common ankle disarticulation procedure was developed by James Syme in 1842.[16,18] It is a weight bearing amputation because the heel pad is swung under the tibia and fibula and attached (Fig. 4.6). The heel flap is securely anchored to the distal end of the tibia and fibula and stabilized after skin closure, either with tape or a rigid dressing until the heel pad has adhered securely. An unstable heel pad (Fig. 4.6b) interferes with good prosthetic fit, can be painful, and limits weight bearing capabilities. In Syme's procedure, muscles and tendons that cross the joint are pulled down, divided, and allowed to retract. The procedure is usually performed in a single stage except in the presence of forefoot infection. During the Korean War, many soldiers received severe injuries to their feet by stepping on bamboo spikes that had been smeared with human excrement. Because these wounds did not heal, Syme amputations were performed in two stages. During the first stage, the foot was removed, the heel pad was brought under the tibia and sutured, and drains were inserted for antibiotic irrigation. In the second stage, done several weeks later when all signs of infection were gone, the malleoli were removed to the joint surface and the skin around the heel pad trimmed carefully to allow for closure without tension. The residual limb was then wrapped in plaster for healing. A modified one-stage Syme amputation was reported by Sarmiento.[19,20] Before closing, the metaphyseal flare of the distal tibia is removed and the distal end of the fibula is beveled to reduce the bulbous end by about one third while retaining the end-bearing feature of the limb (Fig. 4.7). Postoperatively, the limb is placed in a

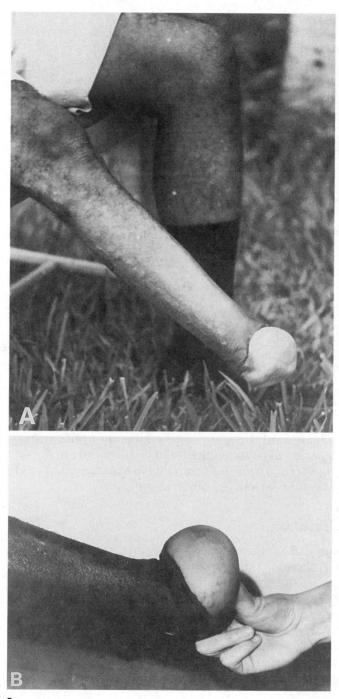

FIGURE 4.6

(*A*) Residual limb after a Syme amputation. (*B*) Unstable heel pad on a Syme residual limb.

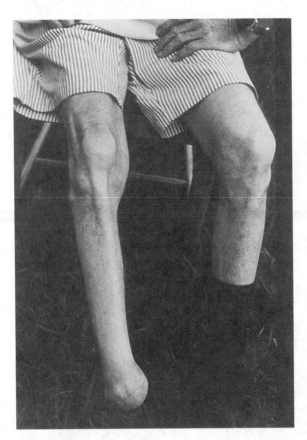

FIGURE 4.7
Residual limb after a modified Syme amputation.

plaster cast until the end pad has adhered properly. In all Syme amputations, care must be taken to maintain the blood supply to the end pad to allow proper healing. Generally, skin flaps either are not trimmed or are minimally trimmed to prevent damage to the blood supply.

Knee Disarticulations

Knee disarticulation is a relatively uncommon amputation in adults. Although it provides a long muscular lever arm for prosthetic mobility, the bulbous end created by the femoral condyles leaves a cosmetically poor residual limb. Knee disarticulations are generally performed for trauma and usually where not enough tibia is left (less than 4 centimeters) for a functional transtibial amputation. It is occasionally performed on elderly individuals with lower limb ischemia who are not considered candidates for prosthetic ambulation since adequate circulation to allow healing at the knee disarticulation level will also allow healing at the high transtibial level. Surgical approaches vary according to anticipated function. The most common technique uses skin flaps of equal length, either sagittal or anterior-posterior, to provide a soft tissue envelope for the distal femur.[21] The envelope is created from the gastrocnemius, hamstring, and patella tendons and part of the knee joint capsule to provide an interface between residual limb and socket to absorb some of the shear forces generated

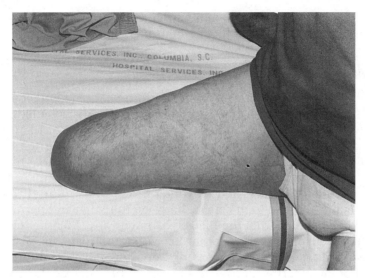

FIGURE 4.8
Residual limb after a modified knee disarticulation.

in walking. The cruciate ligaments are removed; the tibial attachment of the patella ligament is also removed and attached to the remains of the cruciate ligaments. The patella remains in the notch between the femoral condyles out of the weight bearing plane. A more cosmetic prosthetic socket can be used if the distal femur is modified to reduce the bulky distal end. One technique involves resecting the lateral, medial, and posterior flares.[22] Burgess advocated shortening the femur by removing the distal condyles; however, this procedure also removes the suspension assist of the femoral condyles and may require a prosthesis with proximal suspension, particularly as the residual limb atrophies and matures.[23,24] Figure 4.8 shows a residual limb after knee disarticulation.

Hip Disarticulation

Hip disarticulation is a surgical procedure usually performed either for malignancy of the hip or thigh that is not treatable by other means or for severe trauma. On rare occasions it may be used to correct a severe congenital deformity. Boyd's technique, the most commonly used, involves dissecting along fascial planes and dividing the muscles at their pelvic origins or femoral insertion. Closure without tension is permitted because all muscles have been removed except for the large gluteal flap that cushions the distal torso. The incision begins at the anterosuperior iliac spine and curves distally and medially to a point about 5 centimeters below the adductor muscle origins. The incision continues posteriorly around the thigh to the ischial tuberosity, then to the greater trochanter, then continues again to the anterior superior iliac spine. The muscles of the lower leg are detached at their origin, vessels and nerves are ligated, and the remaining gluteal flap is brought anteriorly with the gluteal muscles sutured to the pectineus and origin of the adductors. The anterior position of the scar is distant from the lateral and terminal pressure areas reducing the chance of wound contamination by fecal matter. A firm supporting compression dressing is applied to control edema and postoperative pain.[17,25,26]

Transpelvic Disarticulation (Hemipelvectomy)

This type of amputation is usually performed for malignancy of the hip or pelvis or for severe trauma. It is similar to the hip disarticulation except that this surgical procedure includes removal of all or part of the ilium. The client is placed in a semilateral position on the side opposite the lesion to allow the abdominal contents to move away from the surgical site. The procedure is done in three stages, anterior, perineal, and posterior. The incision is started above the inguinal ligament and extended posteriorly to the iliac crest, then across the pubic tubercle to the crease between the thigh and perineum. The posterior incision extends from the iliac crest downward. An anterior convexity is made as the incision extends anterior to the greater trochanter and comes around the posterior aspect of the upper thigh or along the gluteal fold to meet the lower end of the anterior incision at the ischial tuberosity. The ipsilateral abdominal musculature is sectioned and the peritoneum and attached ureter are pushed medially. The pelvis is usually separated at the pubic symphysis and the ilium is divided between the middle and posterior thirds of the crest or at the sacroiliac joint depending on the site of pathology. The gluteus maximus is reflected with the skin flaps and sutured to the lateral or anterior abdominal musculature (Fig. 4.9). The skin is closed and the residual area wrapped with a compression dressing.[17,26]

SUMMARY

The PT and PTA must understand the basic procedures in amputation surgery to work effectively with the postsurgical client and to provide guidance for proper residual limb management. When possible, clinicians are encouraged to read the operative report to note any unusual findings or surgical variations. Observing surgery is also instructive.

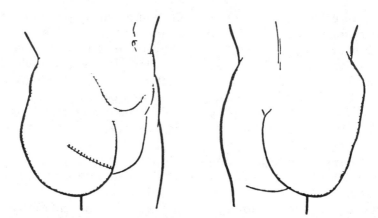

FIGURE 4.9
Diagram of the residual limb after hip disarticulation.

GLOSSARY

Disarticulation	Amputation through a joint.
Flap	A piece of partially detached tissue, usually including skin and underlying muscles and vessels.
Myodesis	The anchoring of muscles to bone when closing an amputation.
Myoplasty	Suturing posterior and anterior compartment muscles together over the end of the bone in an amputation.
Neuroma	Any type of tumor composed of nerve cells identified by the specific part of the nerve that is involved. Amputation neuroma is formed by the cut ends of peripheral nerves.
Patency	A state of being open.
Revascularization	Reestablishing patency of circulation to a part.
Transfemoral	Through the femur.
Transpelvic	Through the pelvis.
Transtibial	Through the tibia.

REFERENCES

1. McCollum, PT, and Walker, MA: Major limb amputation for end-stage peripheral vascular disease: Level selection and alternative options. In Bowker, JH, and Michael, JW (eds.): Atlas of Limb Prosthetics, ed 2. Mosby-Year Book, St. Louis, 1992, pp 25–38.
2. Bowker, JH, Sanders, R, Helfet, D, et al: The choice between limb salvage and amputation. In Bowker, JH, and Michael, JW (eds.): Atlas of Limb Prosthetics, ed 2. Mosby-Year Book, St. Louis, 1992, pp 17–24.
3. Moore, TJ: Planning for optimal function in amputation surgery. In Bowker, JH, and Michael, JW (eds.): Atlas of Limb Prosthetics, ed 2. Mosby-Year Book, St. Louis, 1992, pp 59–66.
4. Bowker, JH, Goldberg, B, and Poonekar, PD: Transtibial amputation. In Bowker, JH, and Michael, JW (eds.): Atlas of Limb Prosthetics, ed 2. Mosby-Year Book, St. Louis, 1992, pp 429–452.
5. Sarmiento, A, and Warren, WD: A re-evaluation of lower extremity amputations. Surg Gynecol Obstet 129:799–802, 1969.
6. Dormandy, J, Belcher, G, Broos, P, et al: Prospective study of 713 below-knee amputations for ischaemia and the effects of a prostacyclin analogue on healing. Br J Surg 81:333–37, 1994.
7. McCollough, NC III, Harris, AR, and Hampton, FL: Below knee amputation. In Bowker, JH, and Michael, JW (eds.): Atlas of Limb Prosthetics. Mosby-Year Book, St. Louis, 1981, pp 341–368.
8. Epps, CH, Jr: Amputation of the lower limb. In Evarts, CM (ed.): Surgery of the Musculoskeletal System, ed 2. Churchill Livingstone, New York, 1990, pp 4(12):83–122.
9. Moore, TJ: Amputations of the lower extremity. In Chapman, M (ed.): Operative Orthopaedics. JB Lippincott, Philadelphia, 1988, pp 603–618.
10. Gonzalez, EG, Corcoran, PJ, and Reyes, RL: Energy expenditure in below-knee amputees: Correlation with stump length. Arch Phys Med Rehabil 55:111–119, 1974.
11. Marsden, FW: Amputation: Surgical technique and postoperative management. Aust N Z J Surg 47:384–392, 1977.
12. Burgess, EM: The below-knee amputation. Bull Prosthet Res 10:19–25, 1988.
13. Bohne, WHO: Above the knee amputation. In Atlas of Amputation Surgery. Thieme Medical Publishers, New York, 1987, pp 86–90.
14. Burgess, E: Knee disarticulation and above-knee amputation. In Moore, W, and Malone, J (eds.): Lower Extremity Amputation. W B Saunders, Philadelphia, 1989, pp 132–146.
15. Harris, WR: Principles of amputation surgery. In Kostuik, JP (ed.): Amputation Surgery and Rehabilitation: The Toronto experience. Churchill Livingstone, New York, 1981, pp 37–50.

16. Gottschalk, F: Transfemoral amputation. In Bowker, JH, and Michael, JW (eds.): Atlas of Limb Prosthetics, ed 2. Mosby-Year Book, St. Louis, 1992, pp 501–508.

17. Santi, MD, Thoma, BJ, and Chambers, RB: Survivorship of healed partial foot amputations in dysvascular patients. Clin Orthop 292:245–249, 1993.

18. Sanders, GT: Lower Limb Amputations: A Guide to Rehabilitation. F A Davis, Philadelphia, 1986.

19. Wagner, FW, Jr: The Syme ankle disarticulation. In Bowker, JH, and Michael, JW (eds.): Atlas of Limb Prosthetics, ed 2. Mosby-Year Book, St. Louis, 1992, pp 413–422.

20. Sarmiento, A: A modified surgical-prosthetic approach to the Syme's amputation: A follow up report. Clin Orthop 85:11–15, 1972.

21. Sarmiento, A, Gilmer, RE, Jr, and Finnieston, A: A new surgical-prosthetic approach to the Syme's amputation: A preliminary report. Artificial Limbs 10:52–55, 1966.

22. Pinzur, MS: Knee disarticulation: Surgical procedures. In Bowker, JH, and Michael, JW (eds.): Atlas of Limb Prosthetics, 2 ed. Mosby-Year Book, St. Louis, 1992, pp 479–486.

23. Utterback, TD, and Rohren, DW: Knee disarticulation as an amputation level. J Trauma 13:116, 1973.

24. Burgess, EM: Disarticulation of the knee: A modified technique. Arch Surg 112:1250–1255, 1977.

25. Boyd, HB: Anatomic disarticulation of the hip. Surg Gynecol Obstet 84:346–349, 1947.

26. Tooms, RE: Hip disarticulation and transpelvic amputation: Surgical procedures. In Bowker, JH, and Michael, JW (ed.): Atlas of Limb Prosthetics, 2 ed. Mosby-Year Book, St. Louis, 1992, pp 535–538.

chapter five

Postsurgical Management

OBJECTIVES

At the end of this chapter, all students are expected to:

1 Compare the major methods of postoperative residual limb management.[1]

2 Implement a treatment program for a client following lower extremity amputation.
   2.1 Teach proper positioning.
   2.2 Describe and demonstrate proper residual limb bandaging and care.
   2.3 Implement an appropriate program of exercises.
   2.4 Develop an appropriate client education program.

3 Exhibit an undersatnding of the psychosocial and economic effects of amputation on clients of different ages.

In addition, physical therapy students are expected to:

4 Develop an evaluation plan for a client following lower extremity amputation.
   4.1 Discuss the implications of evaluation data.
   4.2 Implement the plan with a simulated client.

5 Establish long-term and short-term goals for a client following lower extremity amputation.

6 Design a preprosthetic treatment program for any individual following lower extremity amputation.

case studies

Diana Magnolia: a 54-year-old woman who had a left transtibial amputation yesterday secondary to diabetic gangrene.

Benny Pearl: a 62-year-old man who had a revision to a right transfemoral amputation yesterday secondary to wound infection of a 1-week-old transtibial amputation. The transtibial amputation resulted from a failed femoral popliteal bypass.

Ha Lee Davis: an 18-year-old man who underwent traumatic right transtibial amputation secondary to a motorcycle accident 2 days ago. He sustained some abrasion on the upper right thigh and a sprained right wrist.

Betty Childs: a 12-year-old girl who underwent a transfemoral amputation secondary to IIB osteogenic sarcoma of the proximal right tibia yesterday.

CASE STUDY ACTIVITIES

All Students:

1 Compare and contrast the different methods of residual limb postoperative care; identify the major advantages and disadvantages of each.
2 Discuss how you expect each person to respond to the amputation.

Physical Therapy Students:

3 Develop an evaluation plan for each of the clients listed above.
4 What evaluation activities could you do on the first visit with each client and which must be delayed? Justify your priorities in relation to the client information given here and in Chapter 2.

Physical Therapist Assistant Students:

5 What factors will affect taking goniometric measurements or performing a manual muscle test?

The earlier the onset of rehabilitation, the greater the potential for success. The longer the delay, the more likely the development of complications such as joint contractures, general debilitation, and a depressed psychological state. The postoperative program can be divided into two phases: (1) the preprosthetic phase, which is the time between surgery and fitting with a definitive prosthesis or until a decision is made not to fit the client; (2) the prosthetic phase, which starts with delivery of a temporary or permanent appliance. The major long term goal is to help the client regain the presurgical level of function whether it is to return to gainful employment with an active recreational life, to be independent in the home and community, or even to be independent in the sheltered environment of a retirement center or nursing home. If the amputation resulted from chronic disease, the goal may be to help the person function at a higher level than was possible immediately before surgery.

Postoperative Dressings

The postoperative dressing protects the incision and residual limb and controls postoperative edema. Edema control is critical because excessive edema in the residual limb compromises healing and causes pain. The postoperative dressing may include: (1) immediate postoperative fitting or rigid dressing; (2) semirigid dressing; (3) controlled environment; or (4) soft dressing.

RIGID DRESSINGS

In the early 1960s, orthopedic surgeons in the United States started experimenting with immediate postoperative prosthetic fitting, a technique developed in Europe that consisted of fitting the client with a plaster prosthetic socket. An attachment at the distal end of the dressing allowed the addition of a foot and pylon for limited weight bearing ambulation (Fig. 5.1).[2-4] Use of immediate postoperative rigid dressings varies greatly. Generally, orthopedic surgeons use the technique more frequently than vascular surgeons. Use of an immediate postoperative prosthesis:

1   Greatly limits the development of postoperative edema, thereby reducing postoperative pain and enhancing wound healing
2   Allows earlier bipedal ambulation with the attachment of a pylon and foot
3   Allows earlier fitting of a definitive prosthesis by reducing the length of time needed to shrink the residual limb[2-5]

However, it also:

1   Requires careful application by individuals knowledgeable about prosthetic principles
2   Requires close supervision during the early healing stage

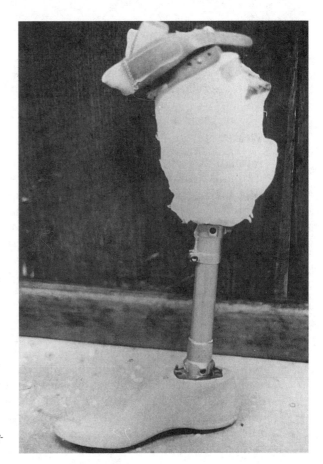

FIGURE 5.1
Rigid postoperative dressing with pylon and prosthetic foot attached.

3   Does not allow daily wound inspection and dressing changes unless the cast has a removable window at the distal end

SEMIRIGID DRESSINGS

Semirigid dressings (SRDs) provide better control of edema than soft dressings, but each has some disadvantage that limits its use. SRDs are made of a paste compound of zinc oxide, gelatin, glycerin, and calamine and are applied in the operating or recovery room.[6,7] The dressing adheres to the skin, eliminating the need for a suspension belt and allowing slight joint movement. SRDs have been shown to be more effective than soft dressings in helping reduce postoperative edema.[7] The major disadvantages are that they may loosen with use and are not as rigid as plaster dressings.

Little first reported the use of an air splint to control postoperative edema as well as to aid in early ambulation.[8,9] The air splint is a plastic, double wall bag that is pumped to the desired level of rigidity. The residual limb is covered with an appropriate postoperative dressing and inserted in the bag. Although the air splint allows wound inspection, its constant pressure does not intimately conform to the shape of the residual limb. Because the plastic is hot and humid, it also needs frequent cleaning.

SOFT DRESSINGS

Soft dressings are the oldest method of postsurgical management of the residual limb. Two forms of soft dressings are the elastic wrap and the elastic shrinker. Both are relatively inexpensive, lightweight, readily available, and washable.

Elastic Wrap

Immediately after surgery, the elastic bandage is applied over the postsurgical dressing with moderate compression, preferably using a figure of eight pattern (Fig. 5.2). The soft dressing is probably the most frequently used and is generally indicated in cases of local infection. It is easier to use than rigid or semirigid dressings. Elastic wrap is not as effective in controlling edema as either the rigid or semirigid dressings. Elastic wrap needs frequent rewrapping; movement of the residual limb against the bedclothes, bending and extending the proximal joints, and general body movements cause slippage and wrinkling. Wrinkles in the elastic bandage create uneven pressure on the residual limb that can lead to skin abrasions and breakdown. Covering the finished wrap with a stockinet helps reduce some of the wrinkling; however, careful and frequent rewrapping is the only effective way to prevent complications. Nursing staff, as well as the therapy staff, need to assume responsibility for frequent inspection and re-wrapping of the residual limb while the client is in the hospital. After initial healing has occurred, the client or a family member should learn to apply the wrap properly (see Figs. 5.5 and 5.6). Most elderly individuals with a transfemoral amputation do not have the necessary balance and coordination to wrap effectively. Elastic wraps stretch over time and need replacement. Residual limb wrapping is described later in this chapter.

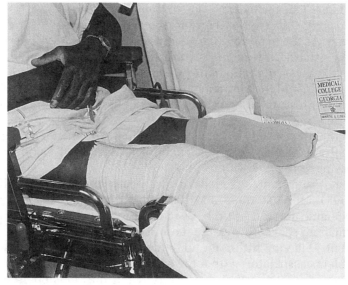

FIGURE 5.2
Postoperative soft dressing includes an elastic wrap over gauze pads.

Shrinkers

Shrinkers are socklike garments made of knitted rubber reinforced cotton; they are conical or cylindrical and come in various sizes (Fig. 5.3). Shrinkers should not be used until after the sutures have been removed and drainage has stopped because the act of donning the shrinker can put excessive and distracting pressures at the distal end of the residual limb and wound drainage will soil the

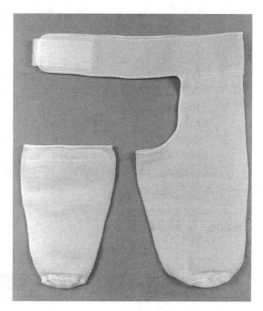

FIGURE 5.3
(*Left*) Transtibial and (*right*) transfemoral residual limb shrinkers. (With permission from May, BJ: Assessment and treatment of individuals following lower extremity amputation. In O'Sullivan, SB and Schmitz, TJ (eds): Physical Rehabilitation: Assessment and Treatment, ed 3. FA Davis, Philadelphia, 1994, p 381.)

shrinker. The shrinker is easy to don and is probably as effective as the elastic wrap, but is less effective than the rigid or semirigid dressing in controlling edema. As the residual limb becomes smaller, new shrinkers must be purchased or the existing shrinker made smaller by sewing an additional seam.

Many vascular surgeons prefer delaying elastic wrapping until the incision has healed and the sutures have been removed. Leaving the residual limb without any pressure wrap allows postoperative edema that causes pain and may interfere with circulation in the many small vessels in the skin and soft tissue. The therapist needs to discuss the benefits of edema control with the surgeon as early as possible and to encourage the use of some form of compression dressing.

Residual limb shrinkage is also necessary before prosthetic fitting. The residual limb must attain a stable size if the first prosthetic socket is to fit for a reasonable amount of time. Because the residual limb continues to shrink after permanent socket fitting, the more stable the residual limb, the longer the socket will fit. Delaying fitting for an extended period of time, however, increases the problems associated with a lower level of mobility. Therefore, a general rule of thumb is to fit the first prosthesis when the incision is well healed and the residual limb has remained stable in size for 2 to 3 weeks. The time between amputation and initial prosthetic fitting varies, but is at least 6 to 8 weeks.

Evaluation

Careful evaluation is an integral part of the management of each client. Evaluation data are obtained continuously throughout this period as the incision heals and the person's tolerance improves. Table 5.1 outlines the typical data needed during a preprosthetic evaluation. The availability of some data depends partly on the treatment of the residual limb by the surgeon.

RANGE OF MOTION

Gross range of motion estimations are adequate for the uninvolved lower extremity and the upper extremities, but specific goniometric measurements are necessary for the amputated extremity. Measurements of hip flexion and extension, abduction, and adduction are taken early in the postoperative phase following transtibial amputation. Measurements of knee flexion and extension are taken, if the dressing allows, after some incisional healing has occurred. Hip flexion, extension, abduction, and adduction range of motion measurements are taken several days after transfemoral amputation when the dressing allows. Measurement of internal and external hip rotation of the transfemoral residual limb is difficult to obtain, and unnecessary if no gross abnormality or pathology is evident. Joint range of motion is monitored throughout the preprosthetic period.

MUSCLE STRENGTH

Gross manual muscle testing of the upper extremities and uninvolved lower extremity is performed early in the postoperative period. Manual muscle testing of the amputated extremity must usually wait until healing has occurred. Although individuals with muscle weakness of the residual limb can be satisfac-

T A B L E 5 . 1 **PREPROSTHETIC EVALUATION GUIDE**

General medical information	Cause of amputation (disease, tumor, trauma, congenital)
	Associated diseases and symptoms (neuropathy, visual disturbances, cardiopulmonary disease, renal failure, congenital anomalies)
	Current physiological state (postsurgical cardiopulmonary status, vital signs, OOB, pain)
	Medications
Skin	Scar (healed, adherent, invaginated, flat)
	Other lesions (size, shape, open, scar tissue)
	Moisture (moist, dry, scaly)
	Sensation (absent, diminshed, hyperesthesia)
	Grafts (location, type, healing)
	Dermatologic lesions (psoriasis, eczema, cysts)
Residual limb length	Bone length (transtibial limbs measured from medial tibial plateau; transfemoral limbs measured from ischial tuberosity or greater trochanter)
	Soft tissue length (note redundant tissue)
Residual limb shape	Cylindrical, conical, bulbous end, or the like
	Abnormalities ("dog ears," adductor roll)
Vascularity (both limbs if amputation cause is vascular)	Pulses (femoral, popliteal, dorsalis, pedis, posterior tibial)
	Color (red, cyanotic)
	Temperature
	Edema (circumference measurement, water displacement measurement, caliper measurement)
	Pain (type, location, duration)
	Trophic changes
Range of motion	Residual limb (specific for remaining joints)
	Other lower extremity (gross for major joints)
Muscle strength	Residual limb (specific for major muscle groups)
	Other extremities (gross for necessary function)
Neurologic	Pain [phantom (differentiate sensation or pain), neuroma, incisional, other causes]
	Neuropathy
	Cognitive status (alert, oriented, confused)
	Emotional status (acceptance, body image)
Functional status	Transfers (bed to chair, to toilet, to car)
	Balance (sitting, standing, reaching, moving)
	Mobility (ancillary support, supervision, closed and open environments, steps, curbs)
	Home and family situation (caregiver, architectural barriers, hazards)
	Activities of daily living (bathing, dressing)
	Instrumental activities of daily living (cooking, cleaning)
Other	Vital signs
	Preamputation status (work, activity level, degree of independence, lifestyle)
	Prosthetic goals (desire for prosthesis, anticipated activity level, lifestyle)
	Financial (available means to pay for prosthesis)
	Prior prosthesis (if bilateral)

torily fitted with a prosthesis, it is desirable for the client to develop at least 4 to 4+ strength in the residual limb. Particular emphasis may be placed on hip extensors and abductors and knee flexors and extensors. The strength of these muscles should be monitored throughout the preprosthetic program.

RESIDUAL LIMB

Circumferential measurements of the residual limb are taken as soon as the dressing allows, then regularly throughout the preprosthetic period. Measurements are made at regular intervals over the length of the residual limb. Circumferential measurements of the transtibial or Syme residual limb are started at the medial tibial plateau and taken every 5 to 8 centimeters depending on the length of the limb. Length is measured from the medial tibial plateau to the end of the bone or the end of the residual limb if there is substantial soft tissue.

Circumferential measurements of the transfemoral or through knee residual limb are started at the ischial tuberosity or the greater trochanter, whichever is more palpable, and taken every 8 to 10 centimeters. Length is measured from the ischial tuberosity or the greater trochanter to the end of the bone. If considerable excess tissue distal to the end of the bone exists, then length measurements are taken to both the end of the bone and the incision line. For accuracy of repeat measurements, exact landmarks are carefully noted. If the ischial tuberosity is used in transfemoral measurements, hip joint position is noted as well. Other information gathered about the residual limb includes its shape (conical, bulbous, redundant tissue), skin condition, and joint proprioception.

PHANTOM LIMB AND PHANTOM PAIN

Most individuals experience phantom sensation following loss of a limb. In its simplest form, the phantom is the feeling of the limb that is no longer there. The phantom sensation, which usually occurs initially immediately after surgery, is often described as a tingling, pressure sensation, or sometimes as a numbness. The distal part of the extremity is most frequently felt although, on occasion, the person feels the whole extremity. The sensation is responsive to external stimuli such as bandaging or rigid dressing; it may dissipate over time or the person may have the sensation throughout life. Phantom sensation may be painless and usually does not interfere with prosthetic rehabilitation. The client must understand that the feeling is quite normal.

Phantom pain, however, is frequently characterized as either a cramping or squeezing sensation, or as a shooting or burning pain. Some clients report all three. Pain may be localized or diffuse; it may be continuous or intermittent and triggered by external stimuli. It may diminish over time or may become a permanent and often disabling condition. In the first 6 months following surgery, phantom pain is related to preoperative limb pain in location and intensity. That relationship does not last, however, and preoperative pain is not believed to be related to long-term phantom pain.[10]

The cause and treatment of phantom sensation and pain are controversial; the literature is replete with studies of these phenomena.[10-15] Melzack[16] suggests that at least 70 percent of individuals have phantom pain following amputation. He believes that clients view the phantom limb as an integral part of themselves regardless of where it is felt in relation to the body. Melzack believes that phantom sensation and pain originate in the cerebrum.

I postulate that the brain contains a neuromatrix, or network of neurons, that, in addition to responding to sensory stimulation, continuously generates a characteristic pattern of impulses indicating that the body is intact and unequivocally one's own.[16]

Melzack refutes the general belief that phantom sensation and pain occur only with acquired amputations after the age of 5 or 6, indicating that all individuals who are missing a limb from any cause, as well as those who lose the use of their limbs through spinal cord injury, feel the missing limbs.

The residual limb should be examined to differentiate phantom pain from any other condition, such as a neuroma. Sometimes, wearing a prosthesis eases the phantom pain. Noninvasive treatments such as ultrasound, icing, transcutaneous electrical nerve stimulator (TENS), or hand massage have been used with varying success. Mild non-narcotic analgesics are of limited value and no particular narcotic analgesic has proven effective. Injection with steroids or local anesthetics has reduced the pain temporarily in the presence of trigger point. Continuous infusion of a regional analgesic postsurgically has been shown to be both effective and ineffective, depending on the amount of medication and the rate of administration.[17-19] Surgical procedures such as chordotomies, rhizotomies, and peripheral neurectomies meet with limited success. Hypnosis is useful in carefully selected clients. The treatment of phantom pain can be very frustrating for both the clinic team and the client.[11-19]

OTHER DATA

The vascular status of the uninvolved lower extremity is documented. Data include condition of the skin, presence of pulses, sensation, temperature, edema, pain on exercise or at rest, presence of wounds, ulceration, or other abnormalities.

Activities of daily living including transfer and ambulatory status are evaluated; equipment and level of assistance needed are documented. Information on the client's home situation, including any constraints or special needs, is valuable in establishing the individual treatment program. Data regarding presurgical activity level and the person's own long range goals are obtained through interview.

The person's apparent emotional status and degree of adjustment are noted. Emotional adjustment and attitude influence the eventual level of rehabilitation and are discussed in detail in Chapter 6. Exploration of the client's suitability and desire for a prosthesis is begun and continues throughout the preprosthetic period. Any other problems that may affect the rehabilitation program and goals are evaluated and documented.

Setting Goals

case studies

Figures 5.4 through 5.7 illustrate the evaluation data for the clients.

CASE STUDY ACTIVITIES

All Students:

1 Would you expect each of the clients to achieve independent mobility with crutches or a walker before prosthetic fitting? Why or why not?

54 y.o. female had L transtibial amputation yesterday secondary to gangrene from diabetic ulcers. Patient has long history of poorly controlled diabetes mellitus. Medications include Insulin, Ampicillin, Darvocet, Xanax. Seen initially at bedside:

S: "My nub hurts and my toes feel like they are cramped."

O: (L) transtibial residual limb wrapped with an elastic wrap over a soft dressing. The wound is clean with little drainage. Posterior flap closure with sutures in place. Circumferential measurements delayed.

Vitals: BP 135/85; pulse 80.

Range of Motion (ROM):
Left knee: Measurements delayed; knee fully extended on bed.
Left hip: Active flexion = 100 degrees; extension (sidelying) = 5 degrees
Abduction/adduction; internal/external rotation = within normal limits
Right ankle: Active dorsiflexion = 5 degrees; passive = 8 degrees
        Active plantar flexion = 22 degrees; passive = 25 degrees
        Active inversion = 15 degrees; passive 20 degrees
        Active eversion = 15 degrees; passive 20 degrees
Right hip & knee active and passive ROM=within normal limits

Muscle Strength:
Both upper extremities grossly within normal limits. Left hip and knee delayed but all musculature grossly active and functional.
Right hip and knee grossly 4+/5 (Good+/Normal)
Right ankle: dorsiflexion 3+/5 (Fair+/Normal);
        plantar flexion (NWB)=4-/5 (Good-/Normal)

Pulmonary Status:
Strong dry cough; has incentive spirometer.

Functional Activities:
Rolls supine to either side independently.
Transfers bed to chair and back with verbal cueing and contact guard.
Propels wheelchair independently but slowly.
Bed to stand with walker with minimal assistance one person.
Stood by side of bed one minute.

Right lower extremity: Evidence of dysvascularity; dry, hairless limb; minimal toenail clubbing; no sores or open areas. Sensation decreased to touch on plantar surface of foot and toes and dorsum of toes.

Emotional and mental: Patient likes to talk and does so almost constantly. However, she does not appear to listen very well, requiring P.T.to repeat instructions. Verbalized concern for returning to home and work.

A: Alert and responsive individual post left transtibial amputation. Currently dependent in transfers, ambulation, wheelchair mobility and care of residual limb but independent in bed mobility.

FIGURE 5.4
Postsurgical evaluation for Diana Magnolia.

    2 Do you expect to fit each of these individuals with an artificial limb? What might affect such a decision?

Physical Therapy Students:

    1 Develop short term and long term goals for each client.
    2 What does each client have to achieve to be a prosthetic candidate?

The preprosthetic period is designed to:

1. Promote a high level of independent function before prosthetic fitting.

62 year old male had right transtibial amputation a week ago secondary to a failed femoral bypass; Revision to transfemoral level yesterday secondary to wound infection. Patient has history of coronary arterial disease. Patient smokes approx. 1 to 1 1/2 packs of cigarettes per day. Medications include: Procardia, Coumadin, Capoten, Darvocet and Lasix. Seen in PT department.

S: "My stump hurts. I don't feel very well."

O: Residual limb wrapped in a soft dressing: appears edematous; chart indicates minimal drainage; anterior flap with sutures in place.

Vitals: BP145/82; pulse 79

(R) hip:	**Active ROM** (PROM not tested)
flexion (Bkly)	15–90 deg
extension (in Thomas position)	−15 deg
abduction	0–20 deg
adduction	0–5 deg

Strength: (patient reluctant to hold against resistance)
Both upper extremities grossly in 3+ to 4/5 (+−G) range.
Left lower extremity grossly in 3+ to 4/5 (+−G) range.
Right hip not tested.

Functional Ability:
Transfer chair to mat and back=minimal assistance of 1 person.
Bed mobility independent except roll to right side or prone (not tested).
Come to sitting with minimal assistance of 1 person.
Pushes own wheelchair.
Stood in parallel bars with verbal assistance only.
Ambulated in parallel bars for 2 laps with contact guard and urging.

A: Alert and responsive individual complaining of pain and fatigue. Currently dependent in coming to sitting, transfers and ambulation.

FIGURE 5.5
Postsurgical evaluation for Benny Pearl.

2. Guide the development of the necessary physical and emotional level for eventual prosthetic fitting.

If the cause of amputation was peripheral vascular disease, a third general goal is to teach the individual proper care of the remaining lower extremity and an understanding of the disease process.

SHORT TERM GOALS

Short term postsurgical goals might include:

1 Reduce or prevent postoperative edema and promote healing of the residual limb.
2 Prevent contractures and other complications.
3 Increase strength in the affected lower extremity.
4 Increase strength in the remaining extremities.
5 Assist with adjustment to the loss of a body part.
7 Regain independence in mobility and self care.
8 Learn proper care of the other extremity.

18 y.o. male underwent traumatic amputation of the right leg 19 cm below the medial tibial condyle secondary to a motorcycle accident two days ago. The drain was removed yesterday and he is referred for evaluation and treatment. Evaluation at bedside.

Patient sustained an avulsion amputation of the right lower extremity in a motorcycle accident. Replantation was not an option because of the level of injury, the traction nature of the injury and the amount of dirt and gravel in the wound. Patient also sustained a severe sprain of the right hand and wrist and multiple contusions but no fractures. Patient was alert and responsive in the emergency room. Medications include: Tylenol and Keflex.

S: "My hand hurts and the pills don't help. They tell me I'll be able to walk with a wooden leg. What will it look like? Will I be able to ride my bike?"

O: Splint with elastic bandage on right hand and wrist. Rigid plaster dressing on residual limb to mid thigh. Appliance for adding pylon and foot in place.

Vitals: BP 120/65; pulse 60

Gross active ROM and muscle strength evaluation of both upper extremities (except right wrist and hand) and the left lower extremity within normal limits. Muscle test right residual limb deferred; gross active ROM of right hip within normal limits. Independent in all bed mobility and transfer activities. Patient can sit and move in bed without difficulty; transfers bed to chair independently. Can stand on left lower extremity by side of bed.

A: Alert and responsive individual who is independent in all bed mobility and transfer activities and is ready for crutch ambulation.

FIGURE 5.6

Postsurgical evaluation for Ha Lee Davis.

12 year old obese white female underwent a transfemoral amputation yesterday secondary to IIB osteogenic sarcoma of the proximal right tibia. Scheduled to start a special program of adjuvant chemotherapy and radiation therapy as an outpatient in about 2 weeks.

Medications include: Tylenol and Vistaril.

S: Crying:"It hurts and I don't feel good."

O: Residual limb wrapped in a rigid dressing secured with a hip spica.

Vitals: BP 118/70; pulse 68

Gross active ROM and muscle strength of both upper extremities and the left lower extremity appear grossly within normal limits although patient was reluctant to participate in therapeutic activities; ROM and strength evaluation of right residual limb deferred. Residual limb reported to be through distal third of the femur. Appears independent in bed mobility. Able to come to sitting at the side of the bed with much urging and transfer into a wheelchair with stand by assistance only. Refused to come to PT department or to stand for other than the transfer. Patient is listless and tires easily. Patient avoided looking at the residual limb or talking about the amputation.

A: Alert but minimally responsive individual who seems to have little energy and is apparently having some difficulty coping with both the disease and amputation.

Social Service Note (pre-op):

Talked with Betty and her grandmother today, primarily to get acquainted. Betty's mother is at home with two younger children. Grandmother and mother take turns being with Betty. Betty lives with mother and grandmother; father died 3 years ago from cancer of the pancreas. Family has applied for medical assistance. Mother is not employed at this time.

FIGURE 5.7

Postsurgical evaluation for Betty Childs.

The success of the rehabilitation program is determined to some extent by the individual's psychological and physiological status and the physical characteristics of the residual limb. The longer the residual limb, the better the potential for successful prosthetic ambulation. A well healed, cylindrical limb with a nonadherent scar (see Fig. 4.1) is easier to fit than one that is conical, short, or scarred or one that has redundant tissue distally or laterally (Fig. 5.8). Factors that might affect attainment of the goals include (1) the client's vascular status; (2) the client's physiological age; (3) diabetes; (4) cardiovascular disease; (5) visual impairment; (6) limitation of joint motion; and (7) muscle weakness. However, care must be taken not to assume that a client with multiple physiological problems cannot achieve a high degree of independent prosthetic function. In the final analysis, a client must take an active part in the rehabilitation program for achievement of rehabilitation goals. If the client does not appear to be motivated, the therapist should try to understand the client's perspective and ensure that the client understands the relationship between the prepros-

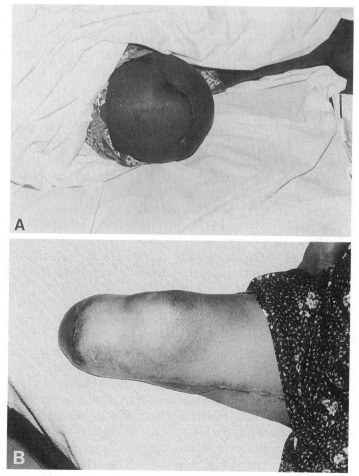

FIGURE 5.8
Short, scarred residual limbs. (*A*) Transfemoral. (*B*) Transtibial.

thetic program and eventual prosthetic rehabilitation. Referral to social or psychological services may be advisable.

Treatment Program

CASE STUDY ACTIVITIES

After reviewing the evaluation data in Figures 5.4 through 5.7 and your short-term goals:

Physical Therapy Students:

1 Establish an initial treatment program for each client.

All Students:

2 What parts of the treatment program are appropriately performed by a physical therapist assistant?
3 Most individuals are discharged from the acute care hospital 5 to 8 days after amputation. What further data do you need to recommend referral for further treatment to an inpatient rehabilitation center? To a home health agency? To an outpatient service?
4 In laboratory sessions practice residual limb bandaging, preprosthetic exercises, and mobility training, role playing each client. How would you vary your approach for each client?

RESIDUAL LIMB CARE

Residual Limb Size

Individuals who have not been fitted with a rigid dressing or a temporary prosthesis use elastic wrap or shrinkers to reduce the size of the residual limb. The client or a member of the family applies the bandage, which is worn 24 hours a day except when the client is bathing.

Removable rigid dressings for transtibial residual limbs are an alternative to the elastic wrap or shrinker. The removable rigid dressing is usually a plaster cast fabricated in the shape of the prosthetic socket and applied after the incision has healed and the sutures have been removed. It is used like a temporary prosthesis with socks and is removed at night and during bathing. The semirigid dressing may also be used throughout the preprosthetic period. A new dressing is applied as residual limb size decreases and the current dressing loosens. Regretfully, there are fewer alternatives for the transfemoral residual limb; rigid dressings and inexpensive temporary prostheses are more difficult to fabricate and elastic wraps or shrinkers are only minimally effective. The semirigid dressing, which is self-suspending and not bulky, may be the most effective alternative. The semirigid dressing, however, is not in general use throughout the United States. Early bipedal mobility affects eventual rehabilitation outcome positively, particularly in the elderly. It may be advisable to fit the individual with a transfemoral amputation with a definitive prosthesis early, then adjust for shrinkage by using additional socks or a liner. Adjustable sockets, as discussed in Chapter 9, may also be advisable. The additional costs involved in early prosthetic fitting and socket replacement may mitigate against early fitting.

Edema in the residual limb is often difficult to control because of complications of diabetes, cardiovascular disease, or hypertension. An intermittent compression unit can be used to reduce edema temporarily. Transfemoral and transtibial sleeves are commercially available.

The residual limb tends to become edematous after bathing as a reaction to the warm water, so bathing at night is recommended. This is particularly important after a prosthesis has been fitted. The elastic bandage, shrinker, or removable rigid dressing is reapplied after bathing. If the person has been fitted with a temporary prosthesis, the residual limb is wrapped at night and any time the prosthesis is not worn. It is equally important that individuals fitted in surgery with a rigid dressing learn bandaging because they can encounter difficulties with edema after they remove the prosthesis at night. Learning proper bandaging is part of the therapy program for all individuals with amputations since most people need to wrap the limb at one time or another.

Skin Care

Proper hygiene and skin care are important. Once the incision is healed and the sutures are removed, the person can bathe normally. The residual limb is treated as any other part of the body; it is kept clean and dry. Individuals with dry skin should use a mild, water-based skin lotion. Care must be taken to avoid abrasions, cuts, and other skin problems. The client is taught to inspect the residual limb with a mirror each night to make sure there are no sores or impending problems, especially in areas not readily visible. If the person has diminished sensation, careful inspection is particularly important.

Clients have been known to apply a variety of "home and folk remedies" to the residual limb. Historically, it was believed that the skin had to be toughened for prosthetic wear by beating it with a bottle wrapped in a towel. Various ointments and lotions have been applied, and residual limbs have been immersed in substances such as vinegar, salt water, and gasoline to harden the skin. Although the skin does need to adjust to the pressures of wearing an artificial limb, no evidence indicates that "toughening" techniques are beneficial. Such methods may actually be harmful because research indicates that soft, pliable skin is better able to cope with stress than tough, dry skin. Client education on proper skin care can reduce the use of home remedies.

The skin of the residual limb may be affected by a variety of dermatologic problems such as eczema, psoriasis, or burns from radiation therapy. Some of these conditions may mitigate against fitting or wrapping. Treatment modalities may include ultraviolet irradiation, whirlpool baths, reflex heating, hyperbaric oxygen, or medication. Care must be taken in using ultraviolet irradiation or heat in the presence of impaired circulation. Whirlpool baths may also not be the treatment of choice since they increase edema. The benefits of whirlpool baths as a cleansing agent for skin problems, infected wounds, or incidence of delayed healing must be balanced against its disadvantages before appropriateness can be determined.

Friction massage, in which layers of skin, subcutaneous tissue, and muscle are moved over underlying tissue, can be used to mobilize adherent scar tissue. The massage is done gently, after the wound is healed and no infection is present. Clients can learn to properly perform a gentle friction massage to mobilize the scar tissue and help decrease the hypersensitivity of the residual limb to touch and pressure. Early handling of the residual limb by the client is an aid to acceptance and is encouraged, particularly for individuals who may be repulsed by the limb.

Residual Limb Wrapping

Most methods of residual limb wrapping incorporate (1) figure of eight or angular turns, (2) anchoring turns around the proximal joint, (3) greater pressure distally, and (4) smooth, wrinkle free application. Clients tend to wrap their own residual limbs in a circular manner, often creating a tourniquet that may compromise healing and foster the development of a bulbous end. Although the client can wrap the transtibial residual limb when sitting, it is virtually impossible to wrap and anchor the transfemoral limb properly while sitting. Many clients cannot balance themselves in the standing position while wrapping the limb. The ends of the bandages should be fastened with tape rather than clips or safety pins that can cut the skin and that may not anchor well. Care should be taken to avoid anchoring the tape to the skin to avoid potential skin abrasions. Elastic bandages that incorporate hook and loop attachments at each end are difficult to roll properly and can cause excessive pressure secondary to the greater bulk of the ends.

A system of wrapping that uses mostly angular or figure of eight turns was developed specifically to meet the needs of the elderly and has been in use for the past 30 years.[20] Figures 5.9 and 5.10 illustrate these techniques.

The Transtibial Residual Limb   Two 4 inch elastic bandages are usually enough to wrap most transtibial residual limbs. Larger residual limbs may require three bandages. The bandages should not be sewn together so that the weave of each bandage can be brought in contraposition to the other to provide more support. To deter development of postsurgical edema as much as possible, a firm even pressure against all soft tissues is desirable. If the incision is placed anteriorly, then an attempt should be made to bring the bandages from posterior to anterior over the distal end to avoid putting a distracting pressure on the incision.

The first bandage is started at either the medial or lateral tibial condyle and is brought diagonally over the anterior surface of the limb to the distal end. One edge of the bandage should just cover the midline of the incision in an anterior/posterior plane. The bandage is continued diagonally over the posterior surface, then back over the beginning turn as an anchor. At this point, there is a choice; the bandage may be brought directly over the beginning point as indicated in step 2, or it may be brought across the front of the residual limb in an "X" design. The latter is particularly useful with long residual limbs, to aid in bandage suspension. An anchoring turn over the distal thigh is made to ensure that the wrap is clear of the patella and is not tight around the distal thigh.

After a single anchoring turn above the knee, the bandage is brought back around the opposite tibial condyle and down to the distal end of the limb. One edge of the bandage should overlap the midline of the incision and the other wrap by at least 1/2 inch to ensure adequate distal end support. The figure of eight pattern is continued as depicted in steps 4 through 7 until the bandage is completed. Care should be taken to cover the residual limb completely with a firm and even pressure. Semicircular turns are made posteriorly to bring the

BELOW—KNEE STUMP BANDAGING

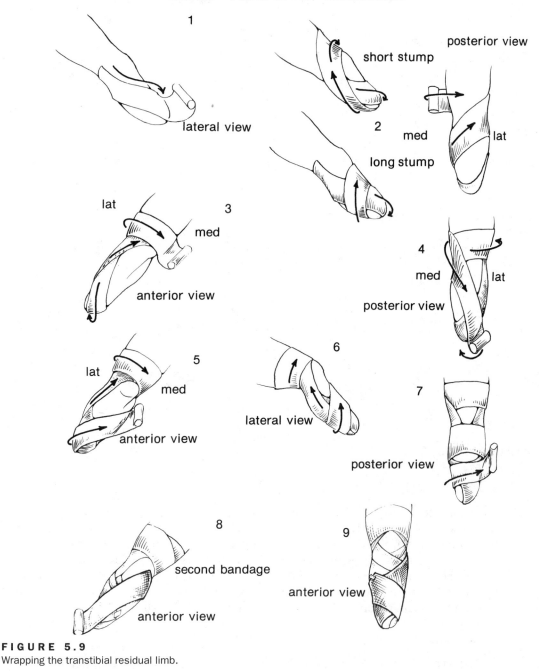

1

lateral view

short stump

posterior view

2

med   lat

long stump

lat   3

med

anterior view

4

med   lat

posterior view

lat   5

med

anterior view

6

lateral view

7

posterior view

8

second bandage

anterior view

9

anterior view

FIGURE 5.9
Wrapping the transtibial residual limb.

bandage in line to cross the anterior surface at an angle. This maneuver provides greater pressure on the posterior soft tissue while distributing pressure anteriorly where the bone is closer to the skin. Each turn should partially overlap other turns, so that the whole residual limb is well covered. The pattern is

ABOVE-KNEE STUMP BANDAGING

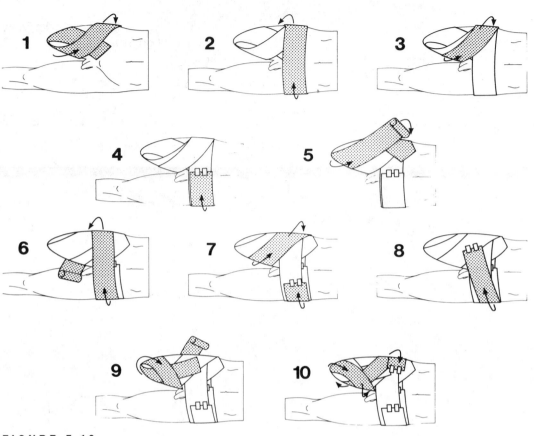

FIGURE 5.10
Wrapping the transfemoral residual limb.

usually from proximal to distal and back to proximal starting at the tibial condyles and covering both condyles as well as the patellar tendon. Usually, the patella is left free to aid in knee motion, although with extremely short residual limbs, it may be necessary to cover the patella for better suspension.

The second bandage is wrapped like the first, except that it is started at the opposite tibial condyle from the first bandage (step 8). Bringing the weave of each bandage in contraposition exerts more even pressure. With both bandages, an effort is made to bring the angular turns across each other rather than in the same direction.

The Transfemoral Residual Limb   For most residual limbs, two 6 inch and one 4 inch bandages will adequately cover the limb. The two 6 inch bandages can be sewn together end to end, taking care not to create a heavy seam; the 4 inch bandage is used by itself. The client is sidelying (Fig. 5.6) to allow a family member or therapist easy access to the residual limb.

The 6 inch bandages are used first. The first bandage is started in the groin and brought diagonally over the anterior surface to the distal lateral corner, around the end of the residual limb, and diagonally up the posterior side to the iliac crest and around the hips in a spica. The bandage is started medially so that the hip wrap will encourage extension. After the turn around the hips, the bandage is wrapped around the proximal portion of the residual limb high in the groin, then back around the hips. Although this is a proximal circular turn, it does not create a tourniquet as long as it is continued around the hips. Going around the medial portion of the residual limb high in the groin ensures coverage of the soft tissue in the adductor area and reduces the possibility of an adductor roll, a complication that can seriously interfere with comfortable prosthetic wear. In most instances, the first bandage ends in the second spica and is anchored with tape.

If the two 6 inch bandages are not sewn together, the second 6 inch bandage is wrapped the same as the first, but is started a bit more laterally. If they are sewn together, the pattern continues with at least two turns coming high in the groin and going around the hips. Any areas not covered by the first bandage must be covered at this time. The second bandage is also anchored in a hip spica after the first figure of eight, and after the second turn high in the groin. Although more of the first two bandages are used to cover the proximal residual limb, care must be taken that no tourniquet is created. Bringing the bandage directly from the proximal medial area into a hip spica helps keep the adductor tissue covered and prevents rolling of the bandage to some degree.

The 4 inch bandage is used to exert the greatest amount of pressure over the middle and distal areas of the residual limb. It is not usually necessary to anchor this bandage around the hips because friction with the already applied bandages and good figure of eight turns provides adequate suspension. The 4 inch bandage is generally started laterally to bring its weave across the weave of previous bandages. Regular figure of eight turns in varied patterns to cover all the residual limb are the most effective.

Bandages are applied with firm pressure from the outset. Elastic bandages can be wrapped directly over a soft postsurgical dressing so that bandaging can begin immediately after surgery. Elastic wrap controls edema more effectively if minimal gauze coverage is used over the residual limb. Several gauze pads placed just over the incision usually provide adequate protection without compromising the effect of the wrap. Care must be taken to avoid any wrinkles or folds that can cause excessive skin pressure particularly over a soft dressing.

Shrinkers The transtibial shrinker is rolled over the residual limb to midthigh and is designed to be self-suspending. Individuals with heavy thighs may need additional suspension using garters or a waist belt. Currently available transfemoral shrinkers incorporate a hip spica that provides good suspension except in obese individuals. Care must be taken that the client understands the importance of proper suspension because any rolling of the edges or slipping of the shrinker can create a tourniquet around the proximal part of the residual limb. Shrinkers are easier to apply than elastic bandages and may be a better alternative, particularly for the transfemoral residual limb. Shrinkers are more expensive to use than elastic wrap; not only is the initial cost greater, but new shrinkers of smaller sizes must be purchased as the residual limb volume decreases. Shrinkers are the best option for transfemoral residual limbs and for individuals who are not able to properly wrap.

POSITIONING

One of the major goals of the early postoperative program is to prevent secondary complications, such as contractures of adjacent joints. Contractures can develop as a result of muscle imbalance or fascial tightness, from a protective withdrawal reflex into hip and knee flexion, from loss of plantar stimulation in extension, or as a result of faulty positioning, such as prolonged sitting. The client should understand the importance of proper positioning and regular exercise in preparing for eventual prosthetic fit and ambulation.

With a transtibial amputation, full range of motion in the hips and knee, particularly in extension, is needed. While sitting, the client can keep the knee extended by using a posterior splint or a board attached to the wheel chair. When supine, the client should avoid placing a pillow under the knee or residual limb to avoid the development of contractures of knee or hip flexion (Fig. 5.11).

A client with a transfemoral amputation needs full range of motion in the hip, particularly in extension and adduction. Prolonged sitting ought to be avoided, if possible, or countered with periods of prone lying and active hip extension. This is particularly important for individuals who have difficulty walking on crutches. Elevation of the residual limb on a pillow following either transfemoral or transtibial amputation can lead to hip flexion contractures and should be avoided (Fig. 5.11*B*). Figure 5.12 depicts general rules of positioning. The early postoperative period is critical in establishing patterns of activity that will aid the client throughout the period of rehabilitation.

CONTRACTURES

Some individuals present with hip or knee flexion contractures. Mild contractures may respond to manual mobilization and active exercises, but it is almost impossible to reduce moderate to severe contractures, especially those involving hip flexion, by manual stretching. Some theorists advocate holding the ex-

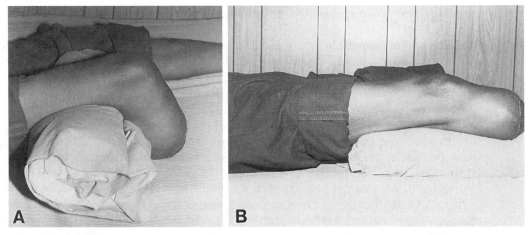

FIGURE 5.11
Improper positioning of the transtibial residual limb.

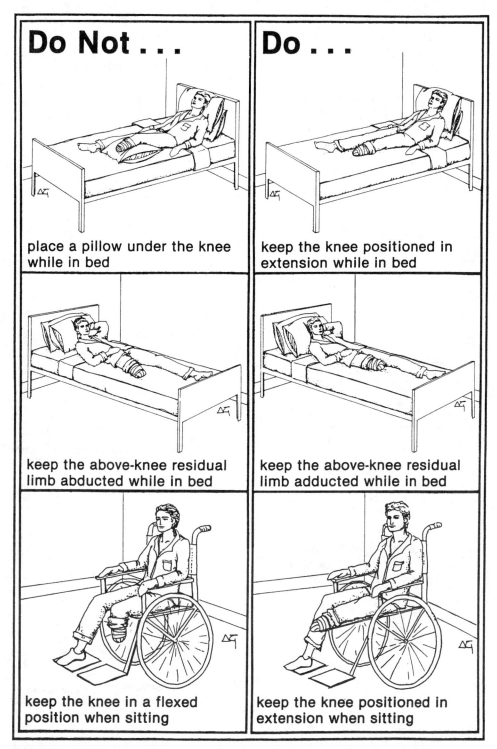

Do Not . . .

place a pillow under the knee while in bed

keep the above-knee residual limb abducted while in bed

keep the knee in a flexed position when sitting

Do . . .

keep the knee positioned in extension while in bed

keep the above-knee residual limb adducted while in bed

keep the knee positioned in extension when sitting

FIGURE 5.12

Correct and incorrect positioning following transtibial and transfemoral amputations.

tremity in a stretched position with weights for a considerable time. Little evidence supports the success of this approach. Active stretching techniques are more effective than passive stretching; hold contract and resisted motion of antagonist muscles may increase range of motion, particularly of the knee. One of the more effective ways of reducing knee flexion contracture is to fit the client with a prosthesis aligned in a manner that stretches the hamstrings with each step (see Chap. 8). Hip flexion contractures are more frequent in individuals with transfemoral amputations. It is difficult to reduce a hip flexion contracture with a transfemoral prosthesis. In some instances, depending on the severity of the contracture and the length of the residual limb, the contracture can be accommodated in the alignment of the prosthesis. A hip or knee flexion contracture of less than 15 degrees is not usually a fitting problem. Prevention, however, is the best treatment for contractures.

EXERCISES

An exercise program is individually designed and includes strengthening, balance, and coordination activities. Exercises may be initiated soon after surgery

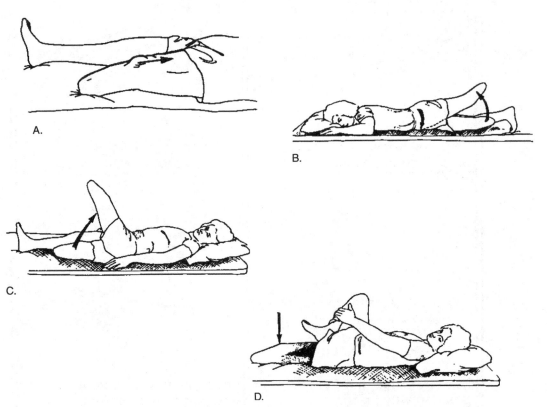

FIGURE 5.13
Exercises for the client following transtibial amputation. (*A*) Quad set. (*B*) Hip extension with knee straight. (*C*) Straight leg raise. (*D*) Extension of the residual limb with the knee of the other leg against the chest. (Adapted from Karacoloff, L (ed): Lower Extremity Amputations. Aspen Publishers and the Rehabilitation Institute of Chicago, Rockville, MD, 1985, with permission.)

if care is taken to avoid stress on the incision or underlying tissue. In some instances, isometric exercise or gentle active exercises within the comfort range may be indicated. Postsurgical dressing, degree of postoperative pain, and healing of the incision determine when resistive exercises for the involved extremity can be started. The postoperative exercise program can take many forms; a home program is desirable. The hip extensors, abductors, knee extensors, and flexors are particularly important for prosthetic ambulation. Figures 5.13 and 5.14 depict a series of exercises particularly well designed to strengthen key muscles around the hip and knee. These exercises can be adapted for a home program because they are simple to perform and require no special equipment. A variety of methods, including the use of elastic bands, provide resistance in the home exercise program (Fig. 5.15).

A general strengthening program that includes the trunk and all extremities is often indicated, particularly for the elderly person who may have been sedentary before surgery. Proprioceptive neuromuscular exercise routines are ben-

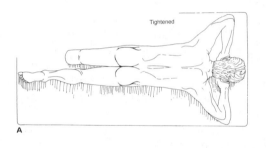

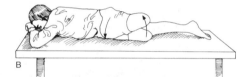

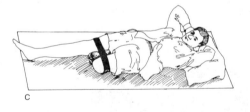

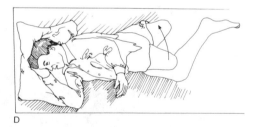

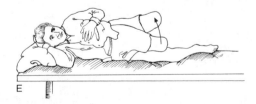

FIGURE 5.14

Exercises for the client following transfemoral amputation. (*A*) Gluteal sets. (*B*) Hip extension. (*C*) Hip abduction against elastic band. (*D*) Hip flexion and extension. (*E*) Hip abduction against gravity. (Adapted from Karacoloff, L (ed): Lower Extremity Amputations. Aspen Publishers and the Rehabilitation Institute of Chicago, Rockville, MD, 1985, with permission.)

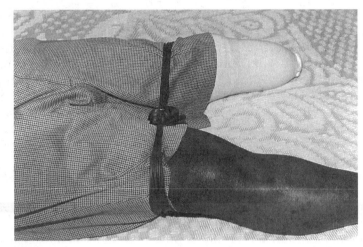
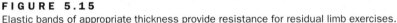

FIGURE 5.15
Elastic bands of appropriate thickness provide resistance for residual limb exercises.

eficial. The exercise program needs to be individually developed and must emphasize those muscles that are most active in prosthetic function. Isometric exercises, such as those depicted in Figures 5.13*D* and 5.14*A*, may be contraindicated in individuals with cardiac disease or hypertension. Both exercises can be modified by having the client actually lift the buttocks off the treatment table in a modified bridging exercise (Fig. 5.16).

A younger, more active client usually does not lose a great deal of muscle strength. Many elderly individuals, however, are relatively sedentary after surgery and need encouragement to develop good strength, coordination, and cardiopulmonary endurance for later ambulation.

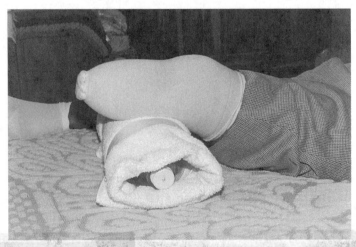

FIGURE 5.16
A bolster or a large plastic soda bottle covered with a bathtowel can be used for modified bridging exercises.

The exercise program is designed for progressive motor control and to increase coordination and function. The client should progress from bed to mat activities using exercises that emphasize coordinated functional mobility. The client's postoperative status is influenced to a great extent by the preoperative activity level, length of time of disability, and other medical problems as well as the side effects of the surgery itself. Because many clients are discharged from the hospital as early as 1 week after surgery, referral to a rehabilitation center or home health agency is important to provide the necessary continuity of care.

MOBILITY

Early mobility is vital to total physiological recovery. The client should resume independent activities as soon as possible. Movement transitions (supine to sitting, sitting to standing) are preliminary to ambulation activities. Care must be taken during early bed and transfer movements to protect the residual limb from trauma. The client must be advised not to push on or slide the residual limb against the bed or chair. The client also needs to be cautioned against spending too much time in any one position to prevent the development of joint contractures or skin breakdowns.

Most individuals with unilateral amputations have little difficulty adjusting to the change in balance point that results from the loss of a limb. Sitting and standing balance activities are a useful part of the early postsurgical program. Upper extremity strengthening exercises with weights or elastic bands are important in preparation for crutch walking. Shoulder depression and elbow extension are particularly necessary to improve the client's ability to lift the body during ambulation. Individuals with bilateral amputations who have one healed residual limb often use that limb as a prop for bed activities and transfers.

Walking is an excellent exercise and useful for independence in daily life. Gait training can start early in the postoperative phase; the person with one intact extremity can become quite independent using a swing through gait on crutches. Many elderly individuals have difficulty learning to crutch walk. Some are afraid; some lack the necessary balance and coordination; and others lack endurance. Some studies have indicated that walking with crutches without a prosthesis requires a greater expenditure of energy than walking with a prosthesis.[22]

Independence in crutch walking is a goal worthy of considerable time in therapy. The individual who can ambulate with crutches develops a greater degree of general fitness than the person who spends most of the time in a wheelchair. Crutch walking is good preparation for prosthetic ambulation; the person who can learn to use crutches will not have difficulty learning to use a prosthesis. The individual who cannot learn to walk with crutches independently, however, may still become very functional with a prosthesis. If ambulation with crutches is not feasible, the individual should be taught to use a walker.

There are advantages and disadvantages to using a walker for support during the preprosthetic period. Certainly, ambulation using a walker is physiologically and psychologically more beneficial than sitting in a wheelchair; however, a walker should be used only if the person cannot learn to walk with crutches. A walker is sturdier than crutches but is awkward to use on stairs. It is sometimes difficult for the person who has used a walker during the pre-prosthetic period to switch to one crutch or cane when fitted with a prosthesis, yet the gait pattern used with a walker is not appropriate with a prosthesis. All clients need to learn some form of mobility without a prosthesis for use at night or when the prosthesis is not worn for some reason.

Temporary Prostheses

Many individuals are not fitted with any type of prosthetic appliance until the residual limb is free from edema and much of the soft tissue has atrophied, a process that can take many months of conscientious limb wrapping and exercises. During this period, the client is limited to a wheelchair or to ambulation with crutches or a walker. Most individuals cannot return to work or participate fully in activities of daily living while waiting for the residual limb to mature. After the client is fitted with a definitive prosthesis, the residual limb continues to change in size and a second prosthesis is often required within the first year. Early fitting with a temporary prosthesis can greatly enhance postsurgical rehabilitation (Figs. 5.17 and 5.18). A temporary prosthesis includes a socket designed and constructed according to regular prosthetic principles and attached to some form of pylon, a foot, and some type of suspension.

A temporary prosthesis can be fitted as soon as the wound has healed. The temporary prosthesis:

1 Shrinks the residual limb more effectively than the elastic wrap
2 Allows earlier bipedal ambulation
3 Provides safer ambulation for individuals who have difficulty walking on crutches or with a walker and one lower extremity
4 Provides a means of evaluating the rehabilitation potential of individuals whose prognosis is questionable
5 Is a positive motivator in that it provides a replacement for the missing part of the body
6 Reduces the need for a complex exercise program because many people can return to full, active daily life
7 Can be used by individuals who may have difficulty paying for a definitive prosthesis

The transtibial temporary socket may be made of plaster or plastic. In all instances, the socket design should follow regular prosthetic princples and should incorporate a prosthetic foot attached to the socket with an aluminum or rigid plastic pipe for proper gait pattern and weight distribution. A crutch tip, more frequently used in the 1960s and 1970s, does not adequately distribute the forces transmitted from the floor to the end of the residual limb and is now contraindicated, particularly for the person with vascular disease. The plaster prosthesis is cheaper to construct and can be changed more frequently. It is not as sturdy as a plastic limb and usually requires the use of crutches for safe ambulation. Depending on the attachments, proper foot socket alignment may also be difficult to obtain if prosthetic components are not used to attach the foot to the socket. Few therapists have been trained in the fabrication of temporary prostheses. Some therapist made sockets are constructed of lightweight thermoplastic materials that can be formed over a positive cast of the residual limb; some are constructed of a fiberglass material formed directly over the

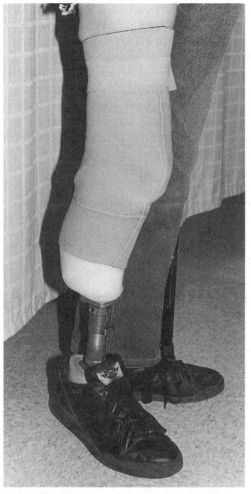

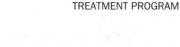

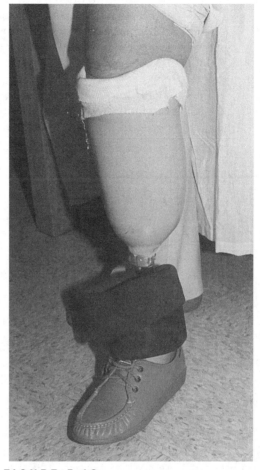

FIGURE 5.17
Temporary transtibial prosthesis. (With permission from May, BJ: Assessment and treatment of individuals following lower extremity amputation. In O'Sullivan, SB and Schmitz, TJ (eds): Physical Rehabilitation: Assessment and Treatment, ed 3. FA Davis, Philadelphia, 1994, p 390.)

FIGURE 5.18
Temporary transtibial prosthesis with sleeve lowered to show socket and pylon. (With permission from May, BJ: Assessment and treatment of individuals following lower extremity amputation. In O'Sullivan, SB and Schmitz, TJ (eds): Physical Rehabilitation: Assessment and Treatment, ed 3. FA Davis, Philadelphia, 1994, p 391.)

residual limb. The prosthesis is usually suspended by a supracondylar cuff to which a waist belt can be added if necessary (see Chap. 7 for discussion of components). The prosthesis is worn with a wool sock of appropriate thickness or ply. The light cotton sock made of stockinet material is considered to be one ply thick. Wool socks generally come in 3 and 5 ply thicknesses (see Chap. 8). When the residual limb has shrunk so much that three 5 ply wool socks are needed to maintain socket fit, a new socket must be constructed.

A temporary prosthesis fabricated by a prosthetist is actually a definitive prosthesis that has not been finished cosmetically. Such prostheses are actually sturdier, allowing regular prosthetic training and ambulation without external support. They are more expensive than prostheses made by a therapist, however, and cannot be changed as readily. Only therapists or other individuals who have received special training in fabrication of temporary prosthetic devices and who have access to appropriate equipment should attempt to construct temporary prostheses. Although it is easier to fabricate a transtibial socket, the use of a temporary prosthesis is important in the rehabilitation of the person with a transfemoral amputation.[21] The temporary prosthesis for transfemoral amputations should incorporate the regular socket, articulated knee joint, foot, and pylon. Suspension may be with a Silesian bandage or pelvic band (see Chap. 7 for details of prosthetic components).

Educating the Client

case studies

As you work with each client, you endeavor to educate the individual on residual limb care. From experience you have learned that the more clearly clients understand the care of their own bodies, the greater their compliance with home programs will be.

CASE STUDY ACTIVITIES

1   Develop a home exercise program for each of the clients. What are the critical concepts you need to include?
2   What teaching methods would work best for each client?

Client education is an integral and ongoing part of the rehabilitation program. Information on the care of the residual limb, proper care of the uninvolved extremity, positioning, exercises, and diet, if the client has diabetes, is necessary if the person is to be a full participant in the rehabilitation program.

Care must be taken not to overwhelm the client with too much information at one time because information overload results in noncompliance. It is more effective to prioritize the information and ask the person to remember a single new thing during each session rather than to try to teach a complex program at one time. It is also important for the program to be tailored to the individual's lifestyle. Involving the client in establishing priorities and setting timetables enhances compliance, as will modifying the program to meet the client's personal goals. The same approach can be used for the home exercise program. After the client has been discharged, either weekly clinic visits or home health supervision throughout the preprosthetic phase can provide a check on home activities, on the condition of the residual limb, and help support the client and family.

Many individuals with vascular disease who lose one leg are concerned about keeping the other leg and therefore are more receptive to learning proper care [see Chap. 2 for components of an education program for individuals with peripheral vascular disease (PVD)]. Ambulation on the remaining extremity is stressful for individuals with PVD who need to be alert for signs of edema, pain, changes in skin color, or temperature. If the person spends considerable time sitting, it may be necessary to elevate the extremity to avoid dependent edema. Intermittent claudication during activity indicates a need to stop the exercise, at least temporarily. The collateral circulation of the remaining extremity is developed slowly through a progressive program of exercises and ambulation. It is important to remember that too little activity may be as harmful as too much.

case studies

Bilateral Amputation

Mr. Canan, 79 years old, lost his right leg below the knee 4 years ago, secondary to vascular insufficiency and diabetes. He was fitted with a prosthesis and became independent with a cane. He was a functional prosthetic user until about 8 months ago, when he began to have problems with his left foot. He continued to wear his prosthesis but did less walking because the foot had become infected. He has just had a left transtibial amputation.

Ms. Darling, 83 years old, has had both legs amputated over the last 4 months because of arteriosclerotic gangrene. The right leg was amputated below the knee and the left leg above the knee. Both residual limbs are now healed and Ms. Darling has been referred to a rehabilitation center for therapy.

CASE STUDY ACTIVITIES

1 How would the short term goals and treatment program for Mr. Canan and Ms. Darling differ from those for the other clients?
2 From the information given, what would be the long term goals in each instance?
3 What data would be important to determine if either individual was a candidate for fitting and training?

The preprosthetic program for the person with bilateral lower extremity amputations is similar to the program developed for someone with a unilateral amputation except for a greater need for balance activities and, of course, ambulation. If the individual was fitted and ambulated after unilateral amputation, the prosthesis is useful for transfer activities and limited standing in the parallel bars for balance. Occasionally, the individual may be able to use the prosthesis with external support to get around the house more easily, particularly for going to the bathroom. Such ambulation generates considerable stress on the residual limb and care must be taken to avoid any skin breakdowns. Fitting with a temporary prosthesis, as previously mentioned, is advisable, particularly if the amputations are at transtibial levels. The higher the initial level of amputation, the more difficult ambulation becomes.

All individuals with bilateral amputations need a wheelchair on a permanent basis. The chair should be as narrow as possible and have removable desk arms and removable leg rests. Amputee wheelchairs with offset rear wheels and no leg rests are not recommended unless the therapist is sure that the person will never be fitted with a prosthesis, even for cosmetic reasons. It is easier to add antitipping devices to the rear of the wheelchair or to attach small weights to the front uprights or under the seat for use when the foot rests are removed.

The preprosthetic program includes mat activities designed to help the person regain a sense of body position and balance, upper extremity and residual limb strengthening exercises, wheelchair transfers, and regular range of motion exercises. With bilateral amputations, individuals spend considerable time sitting and are therefore more apt to develop flexion contractures, particularly around the hip joint. The client should be encouraged to sleep prone if possible, or at least to spend some time in the prone position each day. Therapy also emphasizes range of motion of the residual limb. Some people move about their homes on their knees, the ends of the residual limbs, or the buttocks. Knee pads made of heavy rubber are effective protectors for the residual limbs. Protectors can also be made from foam or felt. Care must be taken to avoid skin breakdown or bursitis around the patella.[22]

Temporary prostheses are of great value in the rehabilitation of individuals with bilateral transtibial amputations. Temporary prostheses are used to evaluate ambulation potential and as an aid to balance and transfer activities. If the individual was initially fitted as a unilateral amputee, the temporary prosthesis will allow some resumption of ambulation. The ambulatory potential of persons with bilateral transfemoral amputations, particularly elderly individuals, is doubtful.

The person with bilateral transfemoral amputations can be fitted with shortened prostheses called "stubbies" (Fig. 5.19). Stubby prostheses have regular sockets, no articulated knee joints or shank, and modified rocker bottoms turned backward to prevent the wearer from falling backward. Because the client's center of gravity is much lower to the ground and the prostheses are nonarticulated, they are relatively easy to use. Stubbies allow the individual with bilateral transfemoral amputations to acquire erect balance and participate in ambulatory activities quickly and with only moderate expenditure of energy. Their acceptance by clients, however, is quite low; some like to use them for activities

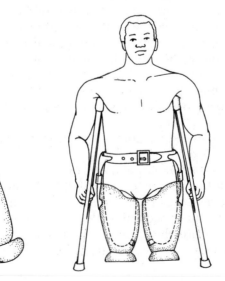

FIGURE 5.19
Stubbies. (With permission from May, BJ: Assessment and treatment of individuals following lower extremity amputation. In O'Sullivan, SB and Schmitz, TJ (eds): Physical Rehabilitation: Assessment and Treatment, ed 3. FA Davis, Philadelphia, 1994, p 392.)

of daily living in the home but rely on a wheelchair outside the home. Although prescribed only rarely, they are most effective for individuals with short residual limbs or those who will not be able to ambulate with regular prostheses.

Nonprosthetic Management

The preprosthetic period is the time to determine the individual's suitability for prosthetic replacement. Not all people with amputations are candidates for a prosthesis, regardless of personal desire. The cost of the prosthesis and the energy demands of prosthetic training require judgment in selecting individuals for fitting. Criteria for prosthetic fitting will be explored in more detail in Chapter 8.

Individuals who are not fitted with a prosthesis can become independent in a wheelchair.[23] The therapy program includes all transfer exercises, activities of daily living, and education in the proper care of the residual limb. Wrapping the residual limb is no longer necessary unless the person is more comfortable with the limb covered. The program emphasizes sitting balance, moving safely in and out of the wheelchair, and other activities to support as independent a lifestyle as the person's physical and psychological condition allows.

SUMMARY

The postsurgical program is very important in the rehabilitation of individuals following amputation. The program emphasizes recovery from surgery, rehabilitation to resume a functional lifestyle, preparation for prosthetic fitting, or evaluation to determine if prosthetic fitting is feasible. The postsurgical program needs to be coordinated among hospital and posthospital team members to ensure continuity of care in a most efficient manner.

GLOSSARY

Bulbous limb	A residual limb with a large round distal end and smaller proximal end.
Conical limb	A residual limb that is smaller circumferentially at the distal end than at the proximal end.
Hyperbaric oxygen	Increasing the oxygen content of the blood by placing a part or the total body in a chamber and increasing the oxygen pressure to a level greater than the atmosphere.
Phantom pain	An unpleasant sensation coming from the absent or desensitized body part. Phantom pain can take many forms.
Phantom sensation	The feeling that the part of the body that has been removed or is desensitized is still present.
Shrinker	A socklike garment made of elasticized material used to reduce edema in a residual limb.
Stump socks	Cotton or wool socks designed to fit over the residual limb and worn with the prosthesis.

REFERENCES

1. May, BJ: Preprosthetic management for lower extremity amputation. In O'Sullivan, SB, and Schmitz, TJ (eds.): Physical Rehabilitation: Assessment and Treatment, ed 3. F A Davis, Philadelphia, 1993, pp 375–395.
2. Burgess, EM: Amputations of the lower extremities. In Nickel, VL (ed.): Orthopedic Rehabilitation. Churchill Livingstone, New York, 1982, p 377.
3. Sarmiento, A, May, BJ, Sinclair, WF, et al: Lower-extremity amputation: The impact of immediate post surgical prosthetic fitting. Clin Orthop 68:22, 1967.
4. Harrington, IJ, Lexier, R, Woods, J, et al: A plaster-pylon technique for below-knee amputation. J Bone Joint Surg (Br) 73:76, 1991.
5. Cutson, TM, Bongiorni, D, Michael, JW, and Kochersberger, G: Early management of elderly dysvascular below-knee amputees. J Prosthet Ortho 6:62–66, 1994.
6. Sterescu, LE: Semi-rigid (Unna) dressing for amputation. Arch Phys Med Rehabil 55:433–434, 1974.
7. MacLean, N, and Fick, GH: The effect of semirigid dressings on below-knee amputations. Phys Ther 74:668–673, 1994.
8. Little, JM: A pneumatic weight bearing prosthesis for below-knee amputees. Lancet 1:271, 1971.
9. Little, JM: The use of air splints as immediate prosthesis after below-knee amputation for vascular insufficiency. Med J Aust 2:870, 1970.
10. Jensen, TS, Krebs, B, Nielsen, J, and Rasmussen, P: Immediate and long-term phantom limb pain in amputees: Incidence, clinical characteristics and relationship to preamputation limb pain. Pain 21:267, 1985.
11. Iacono, RP, Linford, J, and Sandyk, R: Pain management after lower extremity amputation. Neurosurgery 20:496, 1987.
12. Fisher, A, and Meller, Y: Continuous postoperative regional analgesia by nerve sheath block for amputation surgery: A pilot study. Anesth Analg 72:300, 1991.
13. Malawer, MM, Buch, R, Khurana, JS, et al: Postoperative infusional continuous regional analgesia. Clin Orthop 266:227, 1991.
14. Mouratoglou, VM: Amputees and phantom limb pain: A literature review. Physiotherapy Practice 2:177, 1986.
15. Sherman, RA, Ernst, JL, Barja, RH, and Bruno, GM: Phantom pain: A lesson in the necessity for careful clinical research on chronic pain problems. J Rehab Res Dev 25:vii, 1988.
16. Melzack, R: Phantom limbs. Sci Am 266:120, 1992.
17. Malawer, MM, Buch, R, Khurana, JS, et al: Postoperative infusional continuous regional analgesia: A technique for relief of postoperative pain following major extremity surgery. Clin Orthop 266:227–237, 1991.
18. Fisher, A, and Meller, Y: Continuous postoperative regional analgesia by nerve shealth block for amputation surgery—a pilot study. Anesth Anal 72:300–303, 1991.
19. Elizaga, AM, Smith, DG, Sharar, SR, et al: Continuous regional analgesia by intraneural block: Effect on postoperative opiod requirements and phantom limb pain following amputation. J Rehab Res Dev 31:179–187, 1994.
20. May, BJ: Stump bandaging of the lower extremity amputee. Phys Ther 44:808, 1964.
21. Parry, M, and Morrison, JD: Use of the Femurett adjustable prosthesis in the assessment and walking training of new above-knee amputees. Prosthet Ortho Int 13:36, 1989.
22. Perry, J: Gait Analysis: Normal and Pathological Function. Slack, Thorofare, NJ, 1992.
23. Edelstein, J: Special considerations—rehabilitation with prostheses: Functional skills training. In Bowker, JH, and Michael, JW (eds.): Atlas of Limb Prosthetics: Surgical, Prosthetic and Rehabilitation Principles, ed 2. Mosby-Year Book, St. Louis, 1992, pp 721–728.

chapter six

Psychosocial Issues

OBJECTIVES

At the end of this chapter, all students are expected to:

1 Recognize, discuss, and respond appropriately to the anxieties, frustrations, and coping mechanisms of individuals who have had amputations.

2 Compare and contrast the psychosocial responses of individuals with traumatic and acquired amputations, and of older and younger clients.

3 Demonstrate an understanding of the psychosocial effects and financial burdens of amputation on clients of different ages.

4 Describe effective communication mechanisms that enhance the therapeutic relationship with clients, families, and significant others.

case studies

Review the information on Diana Magnolia, Benny Pearl, Ha Lee Davis, and Betty Childs given in Chapter 5.

CASE STUDY ACTIVITIES

1 Compare and contrast the possible emotional responses of Diana Magnolia and Benny Pearl with those of Ha Lee Davis and Betty Childs. What similarities and differences would you expect, and why?

2 What major psychosocial and economical concerns would you anticipate for each of these clients?

3 In laboratory or group sessions, role play the initial and ongoing contacts between the physical therapist (PT), the physical therapist assistant (PTA), and the client.

General Concepts

Many factors determine an individual's psychological response to amputation. Basic personality is a prime consideration. Self confident and secure individuals generally adjust to the loss, whereas timid or self conscious individuals may exhibit greater psychological trauma. Individuals with a strong support system are also less likely to suffer long term psychological distress. Naturally cheerful and easygoing people adjust easily to the loss. For others, joking and laughing may be a mechanism for self deception, calculated to hide fears about possible incapacitating effects of the amputation. Such people may choose tasks or activities that they are not physically able to perform. Prosthetic, social, occupational, and financial factors can either soften or intensify the degree of reaction. Individuals whose jobs or major recreational pursuits have been affected by the loss of the limb may have more difficulty coping than people whose lifestyle is more adaptable to the functional changes imposed by amputation.[1] The level of amputation is not thought to be related to the severity of the reaction.

Many clients are not fully aware of the consequences of amputation, and may fear that other physical limitations will result from the surgery. Fear of impotence or sterility leads some men to make grandiose statements or display reckless behavior to mask that fear.[2] Thorough explanations of the procedures and implications of the amputation by the surgeon or other health care workers may alleviate many of these fears.

Individuals with a history of depression, those who are greatly concerned about their physical appearance, or those who value their independence may exhibit more disabling psychological stress. Rybarczyk et al.[3] found a strong correlation between clinical depression (measured by standardized scale) and social discomfort (described as social contacts during which references to the amputation were made). Twenty-five percent of individuals surveyed were found to be clinically depressed. Clinically depressed individuals tend to perceive themselves as being in poor health and without a strong support system. Individuals who avoid making reference to their amputations or prostheses and who avoid social contacts in the early rehabilitative period may be more likely to become clinically depressed. Nicholas et al.[4] surveyed 94 individuals who had been fitted with a prosthesis and reported that the major social concerns were feeling defenseless and worrying about appearance.

Clients generally dream of themselves as they were before their amputations. This image may be so vivid that they fall as they get up at night and attempt to walk to the bathroom without a prosthesis or crutches. Individuals who have lost a leg through injury may dream about the accident during which they were injured. Such reenactments may lead to insomnia, trembling fits, speech impediments, and difficulty in concentration. Realistic adjustment often comes as the person learns to use the artificial limb. Good predictors for adjustment to the prosthesis are motivation to master the device and desire to return to an active lifestyle.

Psychiatric, psychological, and counseling services are available to help clients cope with the emotional aspects of limb loss (see Chap. 1 for the role of social workers and psychologists). However, most clients do not require such assistance. Understanding and support from family and health care workers are usually adequate.

Stages of Adjustment

Individuals who lose a limb from either disease or trauma may go through several stages of acceptance and adjustment. Bradway et al.[5] suggested four stages of emotional adjustment to amputation.

The first occurs before surgery, when the individual begins to be aware that an amputation may be necessary. It is not unusual to have a client being treated for a vascular ulcer say to a therapist or assistant, "I'm afraid I may lose my foot." The first instinct of health care workers is often to say, "Oh no, no, don't even think that!" Although temporarily reassuring, such a response is not particularly helpful. A more reflecting response ("I can understand your concerns about your foot") may encourage the client to explore feelings about a possible amputation and to raise questions or concerns about prosthetic replacement, pain, financial limitations, and dependency. PTs and PTAs need to create an open and receptive environment and be willing to listen. Grief is the first reaction to the official announcement that an amputation will be necessary.[2,5,6]

The second stage, which occurs immediately after surgery, is usually short. Individuals who have undergone emergency or traumatic amputation may appear euphoric and overly cheerful. Those who had anticipated the amputation may express relief at "having it over with" and being able to start on the rehabilitative process. There may be some expression of grief, as well. The experience may be similar to the death of a loved one. Part of the client's body has been irrevocably lost; the person may feel incomplete and even mourn the lost extremity. Such people may experience insomnia and restlessness and have difficulty concentrating. Little evidence exists, however, that a particular attitude toward the amputation at this stage has any relationship to the eventual level of emotional or functional adjustment.[5]

The third stage occurs as the person becomes involved in the postoperative program and comprehends the permanence of the loss. Some individuals exhibit denial, either through euphoria or withdrawal from social contacts.[7] Younger clients may deny the amputation by trying to exhibit physical capabilities in a wheelchair or on crutches.[8,9] Many individuals mourn the loss of the limb less than the loss of a previous lifestyle. Some may fear the possible loss of a job or the ability to participate in a favorite sport or other activity. Men who lose a limb often fear the loss of sexual capability and potency; some may equate the loss of the limb with castration.[10] In the early stages, the client's grief may alternate with feelings of hopelessness, despondency, bitterness, and anger. The person may experience feelings of internal loss and mutilation. Some state that they would prefer to be dead and wonder why this has happened to them. Clients may be jealous of others who have not suffered as they have; they may blame themselves or the surgeon for the loss. Socially, they may feel lonely, isolated, and objects of pity or horror.[1,2,5]

Throughout this stage, the client may have many questions, so it is important that he or she knows what to expect during the entire process. The steps of rehabilitation and the expectations should be carefully explained, but only when the person asks questions or appears ready to receive the information. Overloading the individual with too much information too early in the process ensures only that the information will not be understood. Individuals with amputations who have made satisfactory adjustments in their lives and have successfully completed rehabilitation can support and encourage newer clients during private or group sessions. Treating the new client in an area with those in later stages of rehabilitation is often helpful, as is showing the client a prosthesis and using films or slides.

Professionals skilled in group dynamics run support groups in rehabilitation centers providing medical or technical advice about diabetes, medications, or peripheral vascular disease. Family and friends are often invited to attend. The atmosphere is nonthreatening so that clients can express their feelings and frustrations. Although support groups are common in rehabilitation settings, they are less common in the community at large. Not all individuals go to rehabilitation centers following amputation surgery; therefore, the PT and PTA need to provide the support in the hospital, in home health care, or in the outpatient center.

The fourth and final stage is related to reintegration into a functional lifestyle. Clients have various attitudes toward the prosthesis. Some are particularly concerned about its appearance, hoping that it will conceal their disability and will give the illusion of an intact body. Others claim to be concerned primarily with restoration of function. When the artificial limb is fitted, the client must face the fact that the natural limb has been irrevocably lost. If individuals with amputations have been told that the prosthesis will replace their own limb, they may have the unrealistic expectation that appearance and function will be as satisfactory as in the nonamputated extremity. Clients who are not candidates for a prosthesis need guidance on community reintegration appropriate to their functional levels.

Many clients make a satisfactory adjustment to the loss of a limb and are reintegrated into a full and active life. Some clients may try to avoid distressing the lost limb through conscious self control or by avoiding thoughts of situations or people that remind them of the lost limb. Some have temper tantrums or manifest irrational resentment. Others may revert to childlike states of helplessness and dependence.

A client may not follow any of the stages or sequences described in this chapter. It is important to remember that the person's preamputation personality and ability to adjust to the demands of everyday life are the greatest determinants of the ability to adjust to amputation. The description of the stages is a guide to help PTs and PTAs understand some of the more common reactions to amputation.

Complete rehabilitation includes preparation of the individual to reenter the community physically and psychologically and preparation of the community for the individual with an amputation. Public education can be used to inform society of the potential of people with amputations in the community and employment. As with other physically challenged individuals, people with amputations need to be accepted and integrated into the community because of their abilities and not their disabilities.

Age Considerations

Psychological distress following any disability increases with age, when all other factors are equal. However, elderly people do not show any greater difficulty in psychological adjustment than the adult population as a whole.[1]

INFANTS AND YOUNG CHILDREN

Shock is the usual parental reaction to the birth of a child with a congenital anomaly or to a child who has an amputation due to injury or tumor. Parents may go through periods of denial and anger and may experience feelings of guilt and shame before accepting their child's amputation. Some parents may be overwhelmed and inconsolable, others may not fully appreciate the implications of disability. Parents of children with acquired amputations may accept the deficit more easily than parents of children with congenital amputations because of the implication of inherited and genetic defect. Rehabilitation team members should be concerned with parental adjustment because parental acceptance of the amputation and the prosthesis will probably correlate with the child's adjustment.

Children are fitted when they are developmentally ready for the prosthesis. A child with an upper extremity loss can be fitted as soon as he or she starts bilateral hand activities, while the child who has lost a lower limb can be fitted as he or she starts to pull to stand. Children usually incorporate the prosthesis into their body image; some refuse to remove the prosthesis for sleep. It is important for the parents and therapists to touch the residual limb normally to indicate their acceptance.

OLDER CHILDREN AND ADOLESCENTS

Regardless of age, the child's emotional reactions must be considered by the rehabilitation team. Too often, detailed discussions about the amputation and postoperative care are conducted only with the parents and the child feels overlooked. The child should be aware of what to expect during anesthesia, surgery, and recovery. Misinformation or distortions should be detected and corrected.

Mourning is normal in the child as well as in the adult. Children, when depressed, are likely to regress to a more infantile level of behavior and must be given the opportunity to express their feelings through play or talk. The young adolescent may grieve over the loss of self-image, whereas the older adolescent may be afraid of rejection and social ostracism. Adolescence is a dynamic phase during which profound hormonal changes lead people to feel sexually attractive and capable of reproduction. Self esteem is very vulnerable at this time. The adolescent may feel inadequate after amputation and may need reassurance from significant others. Contact with other young clients may be quite constructive. Involvement in sports is especially helpful. Reaction to the loss of a limb is affected by the child's previous experiences and by the reaction of family members. Parental reaction profoundly influences the way in which the child copes.

THE ELDERLY CLIENT

The elderly person with a lower extremity amputation is motivated to seek effective rehabilitation services to return to a meaningful lifestyle. The immediate reaction to amputation is no different from that of any other group except that the amputation is usually more anticipated. The reaction depends in part on the severity of preoperative pain and the extent of attempts made to save the limb. Individuals who have suffered considerably may be grateful that pain has ended. Clients who have undergone extensive medical and surgical procedures may experience a sense of failure that such efforts were not successful. If pre-operative attitudes are unrealistically hopeful, postoperative reactions may be more severe. The elderly client should not be led to expect a total cure. Learning to use an artificial limb may be a slow and discouraging ordeal. The client may not express distress or depression when faced with the optimism of others. Sharing and support from other elderly clients can be helpful, as can a realistic attitude by rehabilitation team members.

Stress in the Elderly Client

Elderly individuals are subject to considerable stress from concerns about financial limitations, loss of control over their lives, and fear of becoming dependent. An older person who requires an amputation must often cope with multiple physical problems. Loss is a part of normal aging: loss of physiological capabilities, loss of a spouse or a friend, loss of the self esteem related to one's career or job, and now loss of a limb. It is helpful to give the client as much control over decision making as possible, to provide opportunities for involvement in setting goals, and establishing the sequence of activities.[11] As with any client, PTs and PTAs need to be aware of the stressors affecting clients to assist them to cope by being reflective listeners and enablers.

Cognition and Motivation in the Elderly Client

It is a myth that elderly individuals cannot learn a new skill, that they have difficulty remembering, and that they cannot achieve at the same level as younger individuals. Some older people may have difficulty learning a new skill, but most are fully able to adapt successfully to amputation and to lead a full and normal life. Although some do suffer from dementia, others who are labeled as having dementia because of their confusion in the acute care setting may actually only be responding to medications, metabolic imbalances, infection toxicity, insecurity in a strange environment, or the sequelae of anesthesia. The Mini Mental Status Examination and the Blessed Orientation Memory Test are both reliable and simple evaluations that can be administered by a PT to determine a client's level of orientation and mental function.[12-14] Cognitive dysfunction does not, in and of itself, preclude satisfactory rehabilitation. Understanding the client's cognitive capabilities helps the PT and PTA structure learning experiences appropriately. An individual with cognitive impairment may have difficulty following commands of two or three stages but can follow single stage instructions. For example, saying to a client, "Now you need to reach down and take your foot off the foot plate, then lift the foot plate, then use this little lever to push the footrest out of the way," may be overwhelming because of both the number of instructions and the unfamiliar terminology. On the other hand, the PT or PTA might suggest: "To be able to get up safely from your chair, you need to have these footrests out of the way," while pointing to the footrests. The client might respond by initiating some movements to get the foot off the foot pedal. The PT or PTA can then respond to the client's movements, making additional suggestions as indicated. Using single stage instructions means that only one movement is suggested at one time. Saying "Now that your foot is on the floor, you need to pull the plate up out of your way" (while pointing to the plate), is easier for the client to follow. Using familiar terms and activities can help the cognitively impaired client make connections and respond appropriately. Goal oriented statements may also be clearer to a client. Many activities are almost automatic, such as getting up from a chair, turning in bed, and walking. Most of us have developed particular patterns of movements over the years. The PT and PTA can draw on such patterns by suggesting the movement goal: "Let's sit on the side of the bed."

MOTIVATION AND COMPLIANCE

Motivation and compliance are closely interrelated but compliance is not the same thing as obedience. Everyone is motivated toward some goal. To the extent that the goals of the client and the health care professional are congruent, and that the client performs as the health care professional expects, the client is described as motivated and compliant. If the client has different goals and does not follow the program the health professional has outlined, however, the client is said to be noncompliant. This is why it is important to clarify the client's goals and to organize the rehabilitation program to help the client meet those goals. Kemp[15] has developed a formula of motivation that takes into account the client's wants, beliefs, and rewards as well as the cost of the performance.

$$\text{Motivation} = \frac{\text{Wants} \times \text{Beliefs} \times \text{Rewards}}{\text{Costs}}$$

The client's wants are essentially the same as the client's goals, that is, what the client wants to accomplish. Beliefs relate to what the client thinks of the activity, the future, and the disability. Rewards are the outcomes, pleasures, accomplishments, and positive feelings the client obtains from the activity or program. Finally, the cost stands for the consequences of participation in an activity. Is the activity painful? Does it demand a lot of energy? Does it interfere with other more pleasurable activities?[15] The PT or PTA must consider all the elements of the equation in establishing a rehabilitation program and in planning simple activities such as home exercises.

CAREGIVERS

In most instances the PT and PTA work with a caregiver as well as with a client. The caregiver is an integral part of the team and must be involved in rehabilitation. Caregivers can be members of the family, close friends, neighbors, or paid helpers. Caregivers have their own emotional reactions to the amputation and to the client's illness. Caregiving is a demanding and often tiring activity that can upset family balance and create considerable stress. The PT and PTA need to be open to the needs of the caregiver and to work closely with them. The caregiver's goals, fears, and concerns must be determined. Is the caregiver afraid of handling the client or the residual limb? Is the caregiver resentful of the time demanded by caregiving? What was the relationship between the client and the caregiver before the amputation?

The PT and PTA can provide useful information to the caregiver regarding the disability and prognosis, as well as providing helpful techniques for coping with daily life. Providing time for the caregiver to ask questions and to voice concerns can be an integral part of the therapeutic intervention. Many caregivers, afraid of "doing something wrong," need to develop confidence in their caregiving skills. Effective teaching strategies need to be used with caregivers as well as with clients to ensure a smooth transition into the home program.[16]

SUMMARY

Most people who undergo an amputation eventually adjust to the disability without professional psychiatric intervention. Many PTs and PTAs are not comfortable with emotional or psychological issues related to limb loss. Each health care provider needs to face his or her own feelings about any specific disability, his or her own fears and concerns related to the loss of a limb, and the effects on lifestyle and sexual function. The PT and PTA need to use effective communication techniques in helping each individual reach his or her highest functional potential. Active listening, acceptance, understanding, and openness are key elements to create effective communications.

REFERENCES

1. Racy, JC: Psychological adaptation to amputation. In Bowker, JH, and Michael, JW (eds.): Atlas of Limb Prosthetics: Surgical, Prosthetic, and Rehabilitation Principles, ed 2. Mosby-Year Book, St. Louis, 1992, pp. 707–716.
2. Friedman, LW: The Psychological Rehabilitation of the Amputee. Charles C Thomas, Springfield, IL, 1978.
3. Rybarczyk, BD, Nyenhuis, DL, Nicholas, JJ, et al: Social discomfort and depression in a sample of adults with leg amputations. Arch Phys Med Rehabil 73:1169–1173, 1992.
4. Nicholas, JJ, Robinson, LR, Schulz, R, et al: Problems experienced and perceived by prosthetic patients. Journal of Prosthetics and Orthopedics 5:36–39, 1993.
5. Bradway, JK, Malone, JM, Racy, J, et al: Psychological adaptation to amputation: An overview. Orthotics and Prosthetics 38:46–50, 1984.
6. Parkes, CM, and Napier, MM: Psychiatric sequelae of amputation. Br J Hosp Med 4:610–614, 1970.
7. Parkes, CM: PsychoSocial transitions: Comparison between reactions to loss of a limb and loss of a spouse. Br J Psychiatry 127:204–210, 1975.
8. Brown, PW: Bilateral lower extremity amputation. J Bone Joint Surg 52A:687–700, 1970.
9. Noble, D, Price, D, and Gilder, R, Jr: Psychiatric disturbances following amputation. Am J Psychiatry 110:609–613, 1954.
10. Mourad, M, and Chiu, WS: Marital-sexual adjustment of amputees. Medical Aspects of Human Sexuality. 47–52, February 1974.
11. Jackson-Wyatt, O: Age-related changes in amputee rehabilitation. Topics in Geriatric Rehabilitation 8:1–12, 1992.
12. Schunk, C: Psychological and cognitive considerations. In May, BJ (ed.): Home Health Care and Rehabilitation: Concepts of Care. F A Davis, Philadelphia, 1993, pp. 255–266.
13. Blessed, G, Tominson, BE, and Roth, M: The association between quantitative measures of dementia and of senile change in the cerebral grey matter of elderly patients. Br J Psychiatry 114:797–811, 1968.
14. Folstein, MF, Folstein, SE, and McHugh, P: Minimental state: A practical method for grading the cognitive state of patients for the clinician. J Psychiatr Res 12:189–198, 1975.
15. Kemp,BJ: Motivation, rehabilitation, and aging: A conceptual model. Topics in Geriatric Rehabilitation 3(3):41–51, 1988.
16. May, BJ: Caregivers. In May, BJ (ed): Home Health Care and Rehabilitation: Concepts of Care. F A Davis, Philadelphia, 1993, pp. 269–288.

chapter seven

Prosthetic Components

OBJECTIVES

At the end of this chapter, all students are expected to:

1 Differentiate between endoskeletal and exoskeletal prostheses.

2 Compare and contrast the major types of feet, knee joints, socket designs, and methods of suspension for transfemoral and transtibial prosthetic replacements.

3 Describe major components used in lower extremity disarticulation prostheses.

Physical therapy students are expected to:

4 Make recommendations for prosthetic components for a hypothetical client.

case studies

Our four clients are:

Diana Magnolia: A 58-year-old woman with a transtibial amputation secondary to diabetic gangrene.

Ha Lee Davis: An 18-year-old man with a transtibial amputation secondary to a motorcycle accident.

Benny Pearl: A 72-year-old man with a transfemoral amputation secondary to arteriosclerotic gangrene.

Betty Childs: A 12-year-old girl with a transfemoral amputation secondary to bone cancer.

CASE STUDY ACTIVITIES

1 Discuss the functions of the major components in the transtibial, transfemoral, and disarticulation prostheses.

2 Reflect on the extent to which a person's lifestyle affects prosthetic replacement and selection of components.

3 What components would you select for each of the clients?

General Concepts

The prosthetic prescription may be written by the surgeon who performed the amputation or by the chief of an amputee clinic. Some surgeons may refer clients directly to the prosthetist, leaving the actual selection of components to the prosthetist; others may refer clients to an amputee clinic if there is one locally. In other instances, the physical therapist (PT) working with the client in the postoperative phase in a home health situation, an outpatient clinic, or a rehabilitation facility may determine when the client is ready for a temporary or definitive appliance and may request a prosthetic prescription. The extent to which any PT may be involved in making recommendations for prosthetic replacement depends on the work setting. In the developing health care market, however, every PT must understand the function of major prosthetic components to assist with selection.

Prosthetic Prescription

The prosthesis needs to be comfortable, functional, and cosmetic, usually in that order. If the prosthesis is not comfortable, the client will not wear it; pain and discomfort can be the greatest impediments to successful prosthetic rehabilitation. The prosthesis must also be functional. It must allow the individual to perform desired activities that he or she would not be able to perform without a prosthesis, with the lowest possible expenditure of energy. For most people, a well fitting prosthesis allows a greater range of mobility activities than would be possible on crutches or in a wheelchair. This may not be true for elderly individuals with transfemoral amputations or for those with bilateral amputations. When the energy demands for prosthetic mobility are greater than for mobility without a prosthesis, the prosthesis is rarely worn. Finally, the prosthesis must be as cosmetic as possible. The importance of cosmesis varies with each person. Many older men who wear long pants at all times are not very concerned with appearance, while younger men and most women want to look as normal as possible.

Many factors must be considered in selecting the optimum prosthesis for each client. In an older time, choices were limited. There was one type of socket for each level of amputation, one or two types of feet, a limited number of knee joints, and few choices for suspension. Newer technology and materials have resulted in a plethora of prosthetic components, some very sophisticated and very expensive. An active individual can have different prostheses for sports and for everyday use. Some prosthetic feet adjust to changes in heel height, thus allowing an individual to switch from sports to dress shoes. Prostheses can be made very lightweight to improve function and reduce energy expenditure. A discussion of all available components and materials is well beyond the scope of this book and would probably be outdated soon. Therefore, only the major types of prosthetic components are discussed and the most commonly used items are described. Each PT and PT assistant (PTA) needs to work closely with the local prosthetists to learn the names and configurations of components in use locally.

CLIENT FACTORS

Many client factors affect the selection of components. The client's general health, weight, activity level, motivation, and ability to set realistic goals must be considered. It is important to know the demands that will be placed on the prosthesis and the client's expectations. Concomitantly, the client needs to understand the limitations of the prosthesis. Unfortunately, many people have unrealistic expectations, believing they will be able to walk as they did before the amputation. Although such expectations may be true for healthy, active individuals with unilateral transtibial amputations, they are often not true for elderly individuals with multiple health problems. Unrealistic expectations are a particular problem for individuals whose amputations are at the transfemoral level. Prior prosthetic use may also influence the type of prosthesis prescribed. Clients often do not want to change from a known component to something new. An individual with a second amputation already fitted on one side may need to have the existing prosthesis matched.

RESIDUAL LIMB FACTORS

The length, shape, skin condition, circulation, range of motion, and maturation of the residual limb influence the type of prosthesis. Invaginated scars and poorly placed thick or adherent incisions can affect the choice of suspension and socket. Sometimes different materials can be used to achieve a more comfortable fit in the presence of residual limb problems. The PT can provide information to the prosthetist regarding the location of sensitive areas on the residual limb or other special fitting considerations.

COST

Regretfully, the cost of components may be a determining factor. Third party payers often support only a limited range of components and many clients cannot personally afford the more expensive items. Efforts at cost containment often limit the selection of technologically advanced components that may contribute to a higher level of function. The PT needs to take every opportunity to be involved in component selection and to use his or her knowledge of the client's functional abilities to justify the use of such components. Some prosthetic components require a higher level of maintenance; thus the proximity of the client to prosthetic and treatment facilities may be a factor in the prosthetic prescribed.

PROSTHESES

Lower extremity prostheses include a foot, a knee joint for transfemoral and higher levels, a socket, and a method of suspension. The prosthesis may be endoskeletal or exoskeletal in structure (Fig. 7.1) The endoskeletal prosthesis uses a lightweight metal pylon to connect the foot to the socket (transtibial) or

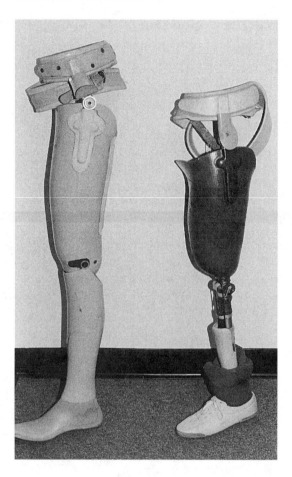

FIGURE 7.1
(*Left*) Exoskeletal transfemoral prosthesis with stance control mechanical knee mechanism. (*Right*) Endoskeletal transfemoral prosthesis with cosmetic cover rolled down.

knee unit (transfemoral). The shank is covered with a foam cover that matches the color and configuration of the other leg. Endoskeletal prostheses use a modular concept in that adjustable components of standardized design and dimensions are readily interchangeable. Through this system, various combinations of components can be tried to find the best combination for a given person. The endoskeletal modular system offers simpler and faster maintenance. It also permits more frequent and easier adjustments of alignment. Socket interchange can be made without destroying the prosthesis. The flexible foam cover improves appearance and can be removed for adjustments when necessary. Adjustable devices are particularly beneficial for children because their growth necessitates frequent changes. Although endoskeletal prostheses are more cosmetic, the cover is not as durable as the exoskeletal devices.

Exoskeletal prosthesis are constructed of wood or rigid polyurethane covered with rigid plastic lamination. The rigidity of the shank makes them more durable and more resistant to external wear than endoskeletal prostheses. Most exoskeletal prostheses are initially less expensive than endoskeletal devices.

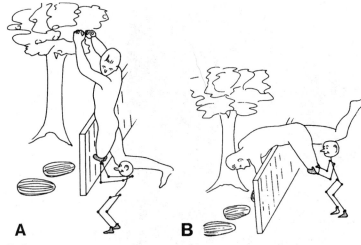

FIGURE 7.2
The prosthesis must (*A*) support the body weight and (*B*) hold the residual limb firmly during all activities. (With permission from Hall CB: Prosthetic socket shape as related to anatomy in lower extremity amputees. Clinical Orthopaedics and Related Research 37, 1964.)

SOCKETS

Socket design varies with the level of amputation and the configurations of the individual residual limb. Specific design considerations are discussed under each major prosthesis. Some general principles of socket design apply to all prostheses. PTs and PTAs should understand basic design principles to evaluate the fit of a prosthesis properly and to perform troubleshooting when clients have pain or exhibit gait deviations.

The prosthetic socket must support body weight and hold the residual limb firmly and comfortably during all activities (Fig. 7.2). Each area of the residual limb tolerates pressure differently, the tissues are selectively loaded so that the greatest weight is borne by pressure-tolerant tissue, such as wide and flat bony areas or tendons, and the least by pressure-sensitive tissue such as nerves that are closer to the skin and to sharp bony prominences. This is accomplished by relief (socket concavity) over pressure sensitive areas and socket convexity over pressure tolerant areas. Additionally, the socket needs to grip the residual limb firmly to reduce movement between the socket and the skin. More movement between the residual limb and socket will make the client less secure during activities and at greater risk for skin abrasions. Total contact between the distal end of the residual limb and the socket is required to aid in proprioceptive feedback and to prevent dependent edema and skin problems.

Sockets are individually constructed for each client from a cast of the client's residual limb. The prosthetist notes the individual characteristics of the residual limb, takes measurements of both the residual limb and the other leg, and makes a cast of the residual limb according to established construction principles. A positive model is made from the cast. The prosthetist modifies the model to improve pressure distribution and socket fit. The socket may be constructed with computer aided design and computer aided manufacture tech-

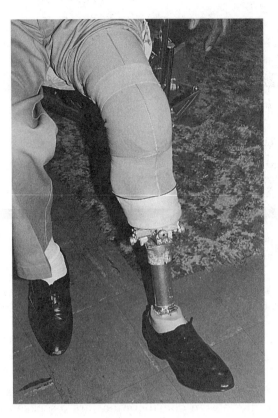

FIGURE 7.3
Transtibial prosthesis on an alignment instrument.

niques (CAD/CAM). The prosthetist uses an electronic scanner to determine the shape of the amputation limb, then fits a test socket to ensure comfort, to provide for appropriate weight bearing, and to stabilize pressures. The prosthetist may also construct the socket using a machine that molds plastic directly over the positive model of the residual limb. The socket is connected to the appropriate components with an alignment instrument between the socket and knee mechanism (transfemoral) or pylon (transtibial) (Fig. 7.3). The prosthetist performs a static alignment with the client standing to set the proper length and to ensure that the components are aligned with each other to maximize comfort and control. Depending on the client's ambulatory ability, dynamic alignment may also be performed at the same time. New clients often need gait training before final dynamic alignment can be set (see Chap. 8).

Ankle/Foot Mechanisms

The prosthetic foot is the foundation of all prostheses except partial foot amputations. It should serve the following functions:

1   Simulate joint motion and muscle activity. The normal foot allows dorsiflexion and plantar flexion, inversion and eversion, and a smooth roll over from heel contact to toe off. All prosthetic feet provide some degree of plantar flexion, but few provide any degree of inversion or eversion.
2   To simulate muscle activity. The anatomic foot and ankle have a complex neuromuscular structure that allows considerable control of mobility activ-

ities such as running, jumping, balancing on narrow surfaces, or standing on one foot. The prosthetic foot substitutes for muscle action primarily through stance phase stability, some variation in plantar flexion, and passive dorsiflexion in swing phase. Various dynamic response or energy conserving feet provide some degree of propulsion in terminal stance.

3 Absorb shock. The foot needs to absorb the forces generated at heel contact while allowing a smooth progression to foot flat and toe off. Prosthetic feet for transtibial or lower levels need to allow flexion of the knee during the early stance phase.

4 Provide a stable base of support. The foot must stabilize the body during the stance phase of gait.

Prosthetic feet can be divided into two major categories, the dynamic response (or energy conserving) type and the nondynamic response type. Feet are manufactured in a wide variety of juvenile and adult sizes. Many have simulated toes.

NONDYNAMIC RESPONSE FEET

Solid Ankle Cushion Heel

The solid ankle cushion heel (SACH) foot is a nonarticulated device with a solid wood or aluminum keel, a sponge rubber heel wedge, and a molded cosmetic forefoot with or without individual toes (Fig. 7.4). Plantar flexion is simulated by compression of the heel wedge that is adjusted to the client's weight and activity level. There is no dorsiflexion, eversion, or inversion. It is the prosthetic foot most used throughout the world.

Single Axis Foot

The single axis foot (Fig. 7.5) allows limited dorsiflexion and plantar flexion by bumpers made of hard rubber; it does not allow mediolateral motion or rotation. At heel contact, the plantar flexion bumper compresses offering a true plantar flexion motion. The rapid foot flat increases knee extension and prosthetic stability on stance. The dorsiflexion bumper, which is a little firmer than the plan-

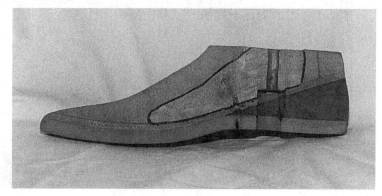

FIGURE 7.4
Cutaway of one type of solid ankle cushion heel (SACH) foot.

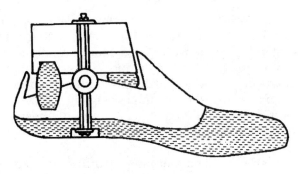

FIGURE 7.5
Schematic of the single axis foot showing the plantar flexion and dorsiflexion
bumpers.

tar flexion bumper, limits dorsiflexion at midstance and terminal stance. The firmness of the bumpers is determined by the client's weight and activity level. Research comparing the function of the SACH and single axis foot reveals little gait difference other than a slightly increased knee stability with the single axis foot.[1-3]

DYNAMIC RESPONSE (ENERGY CONSERVING) FEET

Dynamic response feet were developed initially for clients who wanted to be active and perform such activities as running and jumping.[4] The feet have a flexible keel that increases shock absorption and push off. As clients walk faster or run, they spend more time on the forefoot than the heel, thus increasing the dorsiflexion moment. Dynamic response feet provide this response by using newer designs and materials.

The Seattle Foot[5] (M+IND Corp.) (Fig. 7.6) incorporates a shock absorbing tapered leaf spring that absorbs energy at heel contact and releases it in terminal stance, thereby providing propulsion. The faster the cadence, the more energy is absorbed and then released. The degree of spring also varies with the thickness of the leaf and its material. The degree of spring can be varied to some

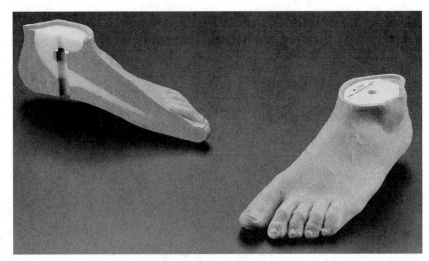

FIGURE 7.6
The Seattle foot. (From the M+IND Corporation, with permission.)

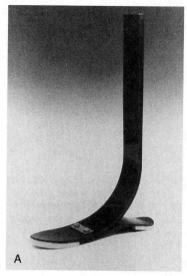
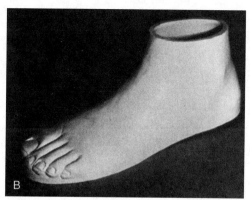

FIGURE 7.7
(*A*) The Flex Foot. (*B*) Cosmetic cover for the Flex Foot. (Copyright Flex Foot, Inc.)

extent according to the client's size, weight, and level of activity.[5,8] The Seattle Light Foot (M+IND Corp.) is a lighter and more streamlined version of the original.

The Flex Foot (Flex Foot Inc.) (Fig. 7.7) is the lightest and springiest of the dynamic feet.[7,8] It is more suitable for active individuals who walk at varying rates of speed. There are several models to accommodate low to high energy outputs. The foot is covered by a foam mold that simulates the normal foot, although many athletes choose to use it without its cosmetic cover.

There are many other dynamic response feet that use a variety of carbon graphite, various plastics, and other materials to provide shock absorption at heel contact and some push off in terminal stance.[4] Several studies have compared dynamic response feet to each other and to the SACH foot.[7-11] Generally, results indicate that clients spend more time on the prosthesis when wearing dynamic response feet; they report having more energy and not tiring as quickly. Athletes also favor dynamic response feet. No significant differences were found in oxygen uptake, however, when the client walked at a self determined pace.[4-11] Table 7.1 outlines the advantages and disadvantages of these feet.

Prostheses for Partial Foot and Ankle Disarticulation

The major functional consequences of single digit, ray, or partial foot amputations are related to loss of push off at terminal stance. Individuals with single-digit or ray amputations may encounter problems with shoe fit but usually do not bother with prosthetic replacement. Shoe fillers of soft foam or cloth can be used. Individuals with transmetatarsal amputations have lost forefoot mobility and support in terminal stance. Additionally, skin irritation can occur at the distal end of the residuum from pressure generated at toe off. A molded shoe

T A B L E 7 . 1 **PROSTHETIC FEET**

Component	Advantages	Disadvantages
Single axis foot	Enhances knee stability for individuals with transfemoral prostheses in which balance and knee control are problematic. Low cost, low maintenance.	Not indicated for transtibial or lower level prostheses or individuals who are active walkers. Faster plantarflexion increases knee extension, slowing push off and gait speed.
SACH Foot	Low cost, low maintenance cosmetic foot that comes in many sizes and heel heights. Can be used with all levels of amputations including Syme's. Most frequently used prosthetic foot.	No propulsion at terminal stance. Cannot vary heel height without changing foot.
Dynamic response feet	Provides propulsion at terminal stance, enhancing the client's ability to walk long distances, run, and jump. Some are light weight and reduce fatigue.	Expensive. Some may provide too much spring for the slow and hesitant walker.

insert can be constructed to provide a firm support surface for terminal stance and to distribute pressure. A full length carbon graphite plate forms the foundation of the toe filler with a molded foot support over it. Very thin carbon graphite plates come in varying densities to accommodate differences in weight and activity level. Some include an arch plate for additional support. The finished molded support includes a filler for the distal part of the shoe.

ANKLE DISARTICULATION (SYME'S)

The ankle disarticulation prosthesis is composed of a socket and a foot; suspension is inherent within the socket because of the configurations of the residual limb.

Sockets

Syme's amputation provides a weight bearing surface at the distal end (see Chap. 4). The socket allows weight bearing at the distal end, along the shaft of the tibia, and a little less at the patella or tendon. It is molded over the shaft of the fibula and the medial flares of the tibia for stabilizing pressure. A window is cut along the medial wall of the socket to allow the bulbous end, created by

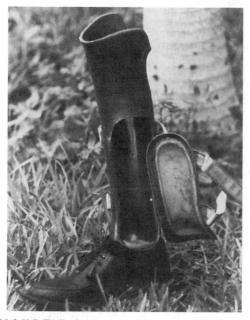

FIGURE 7.8
Conventional Syme prosthesis.

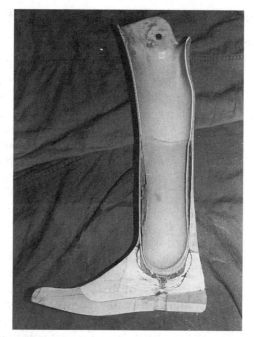

FIGURE 7.9
Cutaway of a closed expandable Syme prosthesis.

the tibial condyles, to slide down to the end bearing part of the prosthetic foot. The window is covered by a panel that fits snugly into the opening and is secured by two straps (Fig. 7.8). The decrease in limb circumference proximal to the bulbous end enables suspension by virtue of the irregular contours of the socket itself. The standard Syme prosthesis is functional but not very cosmetic because of its thick distal end and straps. The medial window also reduces the mechanical strength of the prosthesis.

The closed, expandable socket Syme prosthesis was developed for the modified Syme amputation described in Chapter 4. The smaller distal end created by shaving the malleoli eliminates the need for a window. The prosthesis is fabricated with a liner attached to the inner wall of the socket. This liner is made of flexible plastic and extends from the distal end of the socket to a point where the diameter of the proximal leg equals that of the bulbous end distally. A space is created between the inner socket and the outer laminate. The liner stretches as the end of the residual limb is inserted into the socket. The liner closes around the length of the residuum to maintain total contact and to aid in suspension (Fig. 7.9).

The Foot

Ankle disarticulations result in the loss of all ankle/foot motions. The length of the residual limb precludes the use of most prosthetic feet described in Table 7.1. Some feet, primarily the SACH, have been adapted for use with the ankle disarticulation prosthesis. They provide a place for the distal end of the residual limb.

Prostheses for Transtibial Amputations

THE SOCKET

The patellar tendon bearing (PTB) socket is the standard transtibial socket. It is a laminated plastic socket, fitted with or without a resilient liner (Fig. 7.10). The major weight bearing area is the patellar tendon, an area relatively insensitive to pressure. Some weight is borne over the condylar flares and the distal end of the residual limb. Stabilization is provided by molding the socket over the relatively flat flares of the proximal tibia and the shaft of the fibula, if it is long enough. Areas of relief include the head of the fibula with the peroneal nerve, the distal ends of both the tibia and the fibula, and the sharp crest of the tibia. The proximal posterior wall of the socket is molded to distribute pressure over the soft tissue in the back of the residual limb. It bulges somewhat posteriorly to allow for the muscle bulk. The optimal level for the posterior brim is the popliteal crease, but it must be low enough to allow the client to sit with the knee flexed at least 90 degrees, yet high enough to prevent undue bulging of flesh over the brim. The proximal edge is rounded to prevent sharp pressure on the back of the knee; grooves are provided at the medial and lateral corners for the hamstring tendons. The medial groove is deeper since the semitendinosus muscle inserts more distally than the biceps femoris. The anterior wall reaches to midpatella level and includes the shelf that increases weight bearing on the patellar tendon. The medial and lateral walls reach approximately to the level of the adductor tubercle and control rotation of the residual limb (Fig. 7.11). Total contact at the distal end may be provided by soft foam or by the liner itself.

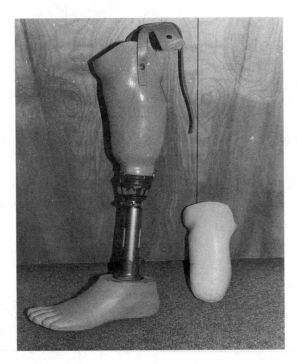

FIGURE 7.10
Patellar tendon bearing socket with liner on side.

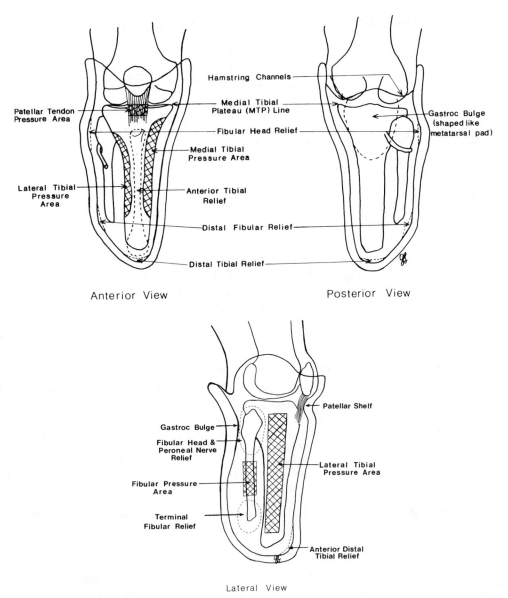

Anterior View

Posterior View

Lateral View

FIGURE 7.11
Pressure and relief areas for the patellar tendon bearing socket prosthesis. (Artist: Gloria Sanders)

LINERS

Most PTB prostheses are constructed with a soft liner made of polyethylene foam or silicone gel that acts as an interface between the residual limb and the hard socket. The liner absorbs some of the compressive and shear forces generated during ambulation. Liners are designed from the same model used in socket construction and fit inside the socket. Liners do not eliminate the need for socks worn directly over the residual limb (see Chap. 8). The liner cushions and protects the residual limb; however, it may deteriorate over time, is not as easy to clean as the socket, and increases bulk around the knee.

Some individuals are fitted without a liner using only the socket and socks. The major advantage is a more intimate fit as pressure and relief can be placed more exactly and with less bulk around the knee. The major disadvantage is that the socket must fit with a greater degree of accuracy and must retain its fit. A liner is the component of choice for clients whose weight fluctuates or who have sensitive or bony residual limbs.[6]

SUSPENSION MECHANISMS

Table 7.2 describes the advantages and disadvantages of the suspension mechanisms.

Supracondylar Cuff

The supracondylar cuff may be made of leather or Dacron webbing. It is attached with studs to the proximal part of the socket in the posteromedial and posterolateral areas (Fig. 7.12). It encircles the thigh just above the femoral condyles and patella. The cuff suspends the prosthesis during swing phase. It is designed to hold the prosthesis over the patella rather than circumferentially around the supracondylar aspect of the thigh.

T A B L E 7 . 2 **PTB SUSPENSION MECHANISMS**

Suspension	Advantages	Disadvantages
Supracondylar cuff	Allows normal knee motion. Easy to don and remove. Relatively inexpensive. Durable and easily replaced.	Does not eliminate all pistoning. No mediolateral knee stability. May interfere with circulation of the distal thigh in obese clients. May cause pinching in distal thigh when sitting.
Waist belt	Provides auxiliary suspension. Some weight bearing on iliac crests.	May be uncomfortable, particularly for obese people. Uneven suspension on swing. Fork strap does not resist knee extension. More difficult to don. Uncosmetic.
Sleeve	Better suspension than all but suction. No circumferential constriction.	Increased perspiration and heat. No mediolateral stability. Not as durable as cuff. More expensive than cuff.
Supracondylar suprapatellar	Improves cosmesis. No circumferential constrictions. Aids in mediolateral stability. Better suspension for short residual limbs.	Enclosed patella can limit kneeling. Difficult to suspend over heavy thighs.
Suction	Reduces pistoning. Minimizes shear forces on residual limb. Does not limit knee flexion.	May be difficult to don. Increased perspiration and heat. Most expensive of all suspensions.

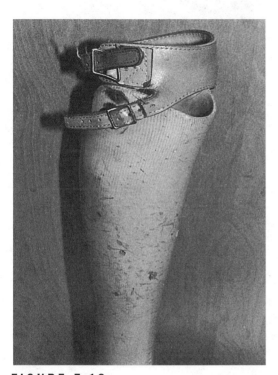

FIGURE 7.12
The supracondylar cuff suspension on well worn prosthesis.

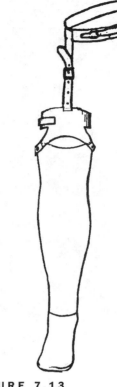

FIGURE 7.13
Waist belt with cuff.

Waist Belt

Individuals with a short residual limb or heavy thighs and those who climb ladders or lift weights may need the additional suspension of a waist belt. A strap, attached to the cuff, buckles to an elastic band that drops from the waist belt on the amputated side. The belt itself is made of cotton webbing and fits around the waist just proximal to the iliac crest (Fig. 7.13).

Sleeve

Latex rubber or neoprene sleeves (Fig. 7.14) come in a variety of sizes and fit over the proximal part of the socket and the distal thigh. The sleeve holds the prosthesis firmly on the residual limb, eliminating pistoning during the swing phase. Suspension occurs secondary to a negative pressure during swing phase and the longitudinal tension in the sleeve itself. To function, the sleeve must terminate above the socks to contact the skin.

Suprapatellar Supracondylar

The proximal brim of the prosthetic socket is extended over the patella and femoral condyles with suspension pressure exerted over the patella and the

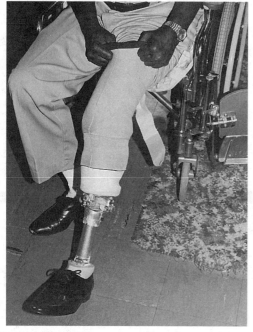

FIGURE 7.14
Sleeve suspension.

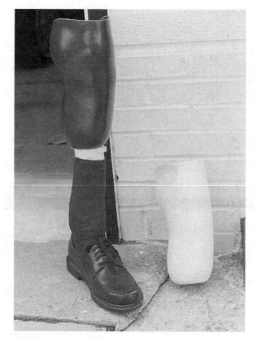

FIGURE 7.15
Suprapatellar supracondylar suspension on a patellar tendon bearing socket prosthesis with liner.

medial femoral condyle (Fig. 7.15). Suprapatellar suspension is created by an indentation of the socket brim over the soft tissue above the patellar. A cup is created for the patella, ensuring that there is no pressure on the patella itself. Pressure over the medial femoral condyle is created by inserting a wedge in the medial portion of the proximal socket. Prostheses with suprapatellar/supracondylar suspension may be referred to as a patellar tendon supracondylar (**PTS**), although the more correct acronym would be **PTBSPSC**.

Suction

The suction socket has a silicone liner worn against the skin. The client places the residual limb with the liner into the socket and attaches it by means of a bolt that locks into the distal end of the socket (Fig. 7.16). Suction is created by the intimate fit of the liner against the skin and the properties of the silicone itself. The liner is soft and is rolled on by the client. The suction socket requires a mature limb that does not change in size.

Thigh Corset

The leather thigh lacer is used mainly when complete mediolateral stability is necessary. The leather corset attaches by metal side bars and hinged knee joints to the socket. It fits around the distal half of the thigh or may extend to the proximal thigh (Fig. 7.17).

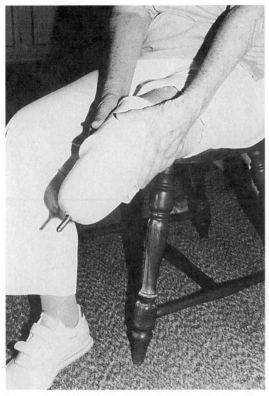

FIGURE 7.16
Donning a transtibial roll on suction socket.

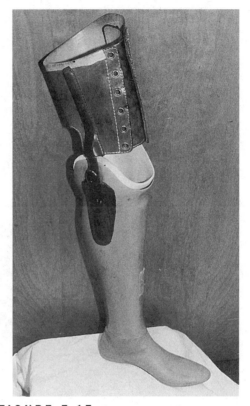

FIGURE 7.17
Thigh corset and a patellar tendon bearing prosthesis.

Prostheses for Transfemoral Amputations

SOCKETS

Two socket designs in general use for transfemoral prostheses are the quadrilateral and ischial containment sockets.

The Quadrilateral Socket

The quadrilateral socket (Fig. 7.18) was developed in the late 1950s and is named for its four walls that each have a specific function. Distally, the socket is contoured to provide total contact for the residual limb. The posterior wall provides the major weight bearing area; the ischial tuberosity and some gluteal muscles rest on top of the wall, which is thicker medially than laterally. Internally, the wall is contoured for the hamstring muscles, while externally, it is flat to prevent rolling in sitting. If the socket is made of rigid plastic, the exterior is padded to absorb sounds and protect clothing. The height of the posterior wall is determined by the position of the ischial tuberosity.

The anterior wall rises about 5 centimeters (about 2 inches) above the height of the posterior wall and medially provides stabilizing pressure to help keep the ischial tuberosity securely on the seat by molding over the femoral triangle. The anterior wall is convex laterally to allow space for the bulk of the rectus femoris muscle.

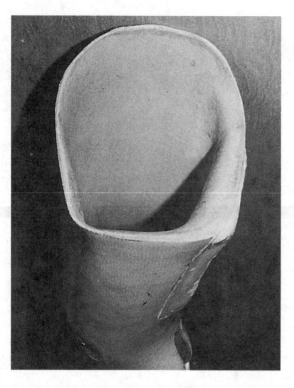

FIGURE 7.18
Transfermoral quadrilateral socket,
viewed from above.

The lateral wall is as high as the anterior wall. For very short residual limbs, the lateral wall is extended proximally above the greater trochanter to increase stability and control. On the inside, the wall inclines medially to set the residual limb in about 10 degrees of adduction. Setting the residual limb in adduction simulates the normal adduction angle of the femur and aids in pelvic control in stance. The lateral wall is contoured to distribute pressure evenly over the lateral side of the residual limb. Relief may be provided distally for the end of the femur and proximally for the greater trochanter.

The medial wall is vertical and parallel to the sagittal plane. The wall prevents medial movement of the residual limb within the socket, especially during stance. A relief channel is built into the corner of the medial and anterior walls for the adductor longus tendon. The medial wall and the posterior wall are the same height. It is sometimes necessary to lower the medial wall a little to prevent undue pressure on the pubic ramus. Figure 7.19 illustrates a cross section of the quadrilateral socket at ischial level showing the relationship of tissues to the wall.

The Ischial Containment Socket

The ischial containment socket (Fig. 7.20) was developed in the late 1980s and early 1990s and is shaped differently from the quadrilateral socket. Improved pelvic control in stance, comfortable weight bearing, and a smoother swing phase are the major objectives of the ischial containment socket. The term **ischial containment** describes its major characteristic. The ischium and the ascending ramus are enclosed within the socket and weight bearing forces are

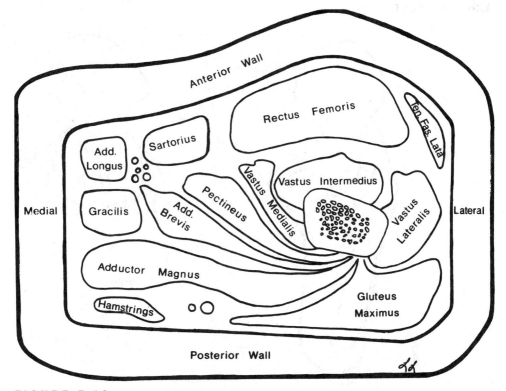

FIGURE 7.19
Cross section through a transfemoral quadrilateral socket at the level of the ischial tuberosity.
(Artist: Lori Leeds)

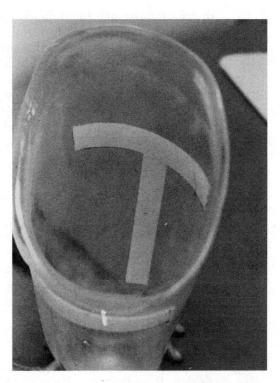

FIGURE 7.20
The ischial containment socket.

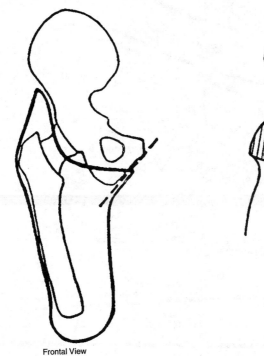
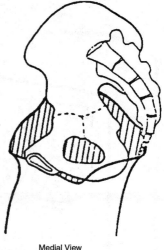

Medial View

Frontal View

FIGURE 7.21
(*Left*) Frontal view of the femur and pelvis in the ischial containment socket. (*Right*) Medial view of the pelvis in the ischial containment socket.

distributed through the medial aspect of the ischium and the ramus as well as surrounding soft tissue. More of the residual limb is contained within the ischial containment socket than in the quadrilateral socket, allowing for greater distribution of weight bearing and stabilizing forces. The narrow mediolateral dimension and molding over the femoral shaft help to keep the ischium and the ramus against the posteromedial wall of the socket and contribute to rotational stability. The lateral wall is extended well over the greater trochanter to add to stance phase stability of the pelvis. The socket is contoured for total contact throughout. Figure 7.21 shows the relationship of the socket walls to the bony structures.

Flexible Sockets

Flexible sockets incorporate a malleable thermoplastic socket supported in some type of rigid or semirigid frame. The frame can be of quadrilateral or ischial containment design; the latter is more frequently used. As in the suction transtibial prosthesis, flexible sockets are best used for individuals with mature residual limbs of at least medium length. Flexible sockets are reported to provide better proprioception, better suspension, and greater comfort.[12-14]

Advantages or Disadvantages

The literature reports no specific advantages or disadvantages for each socket design. If an individual has been using a particular socket successfully, it is beneficial to continue with that design. Schuch,[15] summarizing the recommendations of several authors, suggested that the quadrilateral socket is most successful if the residual limb is long and firm with strong adductor muscles, whereas the ischial containment socket is more successful for short and flabby residual limbs. He further suggested that the ischial containment socket might be more beneficial for very active individuals. Gottschalk et al[16] reported that socket configuration did not affect femoral adduction. Otherwise, it is probably a matter of client and prosthetist preference.

SUSPENSION MECHANISMS

Each of the following suspension methods may be used with any transfemoral socket. The advantages and disadvantages of each method of suspension are outlined in Table 7.3.

Suction

The suction socket (Fig. 7.22) is worn with the residual limb in direct contact with the socket without a sock. The process of donning the socket pushes all the air out the valve hole at the medial distal end of the socket, creating negative pressure within the socket. The valve prevents air from reentering the socket. During the swing phase of gait, negative pressure within the socket augmented by muscle tension holds the socket on the residual limb. Donning the socket (Fig. 7.23) involves putting on a thin sock, standing, and pushing the residual limb into the socket while pulling the sock out through the valve hole. The

T A B L E 7 . 3 **TRANSFEMORAL SUSPENSION MECHANISMS**

Suspension	Advantages	Disadvantages
Suction	Allows full freedom of hip motion. Good proprioceptive feedback through its intimate fit.	Difficulty obtaining good fit. Suction can be lost through perspiration. Potential for skin shear and abrasions. Potential for skin irritation in a closed medium. Requires good balance and coordination for donning.
Silesian bandage	Lightweight additional suspension. Provides some rotational control.	Difficult to keep clean unless it is detachable. Can irritate the waist.
Total elastic suspension	Provides excellent suspension. Adjusts to the size of the individual. Generally comfortable. Adds less weight than the pelvic belt. Provides for rotational control.	Retains body heat, which may lead to skin irritations and discomfort. Wears out easily. Difficult to keep clean.
Pelvic belt	Easy to don. Provides rotational control. Provides mediolateral pelvic stability.	Adds weight to the prosthesis. Is usually not very comfortable.

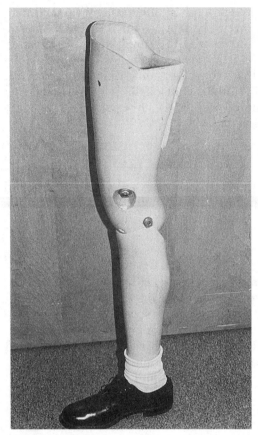

FIGURE 7.22
A transfemoral suction prosthesis with quadrilateral socket and constant friction knee mechanism.

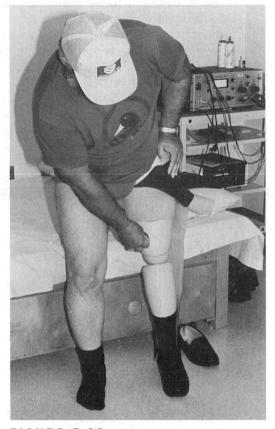

FIGURE 7.23
Donning a transfemoral prosthesis with suction suspension.

client can palpate the end of the residual limb to ensure that it is well into the socket. An alternative method of donning involves spreading a thin layer of lotion over the residual limb. The client then pushes the residual limb fully into the socket and secures the valve. The lotion is absorbed into the skin and suction is maintained.[10]

The flexible socket is simply rolled over the residual limb, then inserted into the supporting frame. Suction provides an intimate suspension and good proprioceptive feedback, and allows full hip motion. It is difficult to maintain adequate suspension with suction alone if limb volume fluctuates or if perspiration accumulates on the residual limb; many clients choose to add an auxiliary suspension.

Suction is indicated for people with firm, mature, and generally smooth residual limbs of medium to long length. A client must have adequate balance and coordination to don the prosthesis properly.

Silesian Bandage

The Silesian bandage is made of a soft webbing strap or leather that is attached to the lateral socket wall, encircles the pelvis, and connects with a strap on the

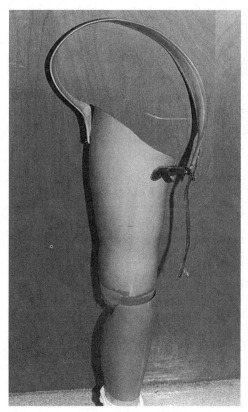

FIGURE 7.24
Silesian band suspension on a transfemoral prosthesis.

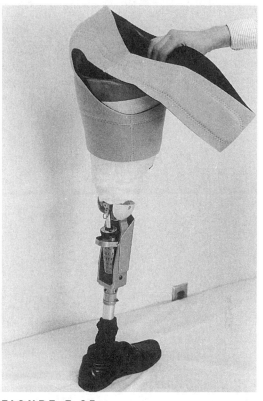

FIGURE 7.25
Total elastic suspension (TES) on transfemoral prosthesis.

anterior wall (Fig. 7.24). The Silesian bandage aids suspension and provides some control of rotation. The bandage is indicated as an auxiliary to suction suspension.

Total Elastic Suspension

The total elastic suspension (TES) is a wide neoprene band lined with nylon tricot material that is similar to the neoprene sleeve of the transtibial prosthesis (Fig. 7.25). The belt fits around the proximal part of the socket and goes around the waist and pelvis to suspend the prosthesis. It can be used with suction or as a primary suspension mechanism.

Pelvic Belt

The pelvic belt (Fig. 7.26) is made of leather and metal and is connected to the prosthesis by a metal or nylon hip joint fastened to the superolateral aspect of the socket. The belt suspends the prosthesis and enables the wearer to don the limb while sitting. It is particularly useful for a client whose weight fluctuates widely. It also provides some mediolateral stability and is useful for individuals with weak hip abductors. It adds weight to the prosthesis and may be uncomfortable against the trunk, particularly in sitting.

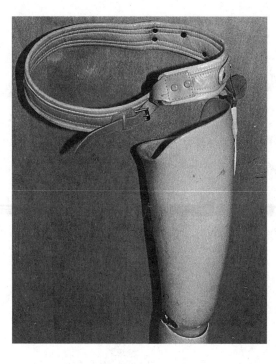

FIGURE 7.26
Pelvic belt suspension.

KNEE MECHANISMS

The prosthetic knee has several functions: (1) to allow sitting, kneeling, and similar activities; (2) to allow a smooth and controlled movement of the shank and foot during swing phase; and (3) to provide stability during stance phase. A wide variety of knee mechanisms are on the market; others are in research and development. It is beyond the scope of this text to review all available knee mechanisms. Representative mechanisms by major function and characteristics are discussed. Readers are encouraged to work with local prosthetists to determine the specific knee mechanisms in use locally.

Knee Control

Knee units may function in stance, in swing, or during both phases of gait. Stability in stance is a function of the way the knee joint is aligned in the prosthesis (alignment stability) and the client's ability to keep the knee in extension (voluntary control). (See Chap. 8 for a discussion of knee control.) The most appropriate knee mechanism is one that requires the least amount of alignment stability, yet offers adequate security in stance. The effort required to initiate swing phase is increased as more alignment stability is built into a prosthesis, thus affecting gait. The amount of alignment stability needed is inversely related to the length and strength of the residual limb. The amount of alignment stability necessary is also determined by the type of knee mechanism used.

The term **stance phase control** refers to the degree of stability when standing on the prosthesis. Stance stability is generally provided by alignment and the voluntary action of the client. In most knee mechanisms, failure to extend the knee fully before heel contact causes the prosthetic knee to flex suddenly when weight is applied. Some knee mechanisms provide some additional stability during stance, particularly if the client does not bring the knee into full extension before putting weight on the prosthesis.

From toe off to heel contact, the shank and foot of the prosthesis swings forward like a modified pendulum. If not controlled by the prosthetic knee, the shank and foot function exactly like a pendulum, coming forward at a rate determined by the force exerted at toe off. For the foot to be in proper position for heel contact, the knee mechanism must exert some control over the rate of knee movement in swing phase. This is referred to as **swing phase control.** Swing phase control may be constant; that is, the foot comes forward at the same rate each step regardless of the speed of gait, or it may be variable responding to the forces generated by the walking speed of the individual.

Knee mechanisms can be classified into two categories: sliding friction and hydraulic. They may be further categorized by the type of control exerted, for example, swing phase or stance phase control. A few knee mechanisms provide for both swing phase and stance phase control. Most knee units are manufactured for both endoskeletal and exoskeletal constructions. Advantages and disadvantages of the major types of knee joints are outlined in Table 7.4.

T A B L E   7 . 4   **KNEE MECHANISMS**

Knee Mechanism	Advantages	Disadvantages
Constant friction	Simple. Durable. Low-maintenance.	Only constant swing phase control. No stance control.
Multiaxis	Varying stability through stance. Shortens shank during swing for better toe clearance. Allows shank to rotate under knee when sitting.	Increased weight and bulk. Complex mechanism, less durable.
Pneumatic control	More responsive to changes in walking speed than constant friction.	Higher cost. Requires more maintenance. Heavier.
Extension aids	Increases speed of terminal extension. Used with many sliding friction knee mechanisms.	Constant rate of extension.
Sliding friction stance control	Braking mechanism if weight applied with knee flexed 0–20 degrees. Helpful to slower clients.	Requires regular maintenance. Not very responsive for active walker.
Manual lock	Total stability in stance phase.	No swing phase flexion, resulting in stiff knee gait.
Hydraulic swing control	Responds to changing gait speeds.	Higher cost than any other unit. Heavy. May need more maintenance.
Hydraulic swing and stance control	Responds to changing gait speeds. Has a braking mechanism for stance phase control.	Higher cost than any other unit. Heavy. May need more maintenance.

Sliding Friction Knee Mechanisms

The sliding friction knee joint category includes all mechanisms that do not have hydraulic units. Knee joints may have one or more axis of motion. Units with one axis of motion are referred to as **single axis knee joints,** others, as multiaxis knee joints.

The constant friction knee (see Fig. 7.22) is a single axis knee that provides constant swing phase control. Some friction is set into the mechanism by adjusting two small screws in front or back of the knee mechanism. The rate stays the same regardless of the speed of gait. It does not provide any stance phase control. It is one of the oldest knee mechanisms in use.

Multiaxis knee joints are usually four-bar linkage systems. They are polycentric axis knees with the changing knee axes providing some swing phase control by shortening the shank during flexion to allow for better toe clearance. They offer some stance phase control by varying stability through the different axes. They are complex mechanically and are used primarily for knee disarticulation prostheses or short transfemoral limbs.

Pneumatic control knee mechanisms use an air filled cylinder housed within the upper part of the shank to provide variable swing phase control. Knee flexion forces air through a cylinder, then through a port that can be adjusted in size. The smaller the opening, the more resistance to swing phase. The amount of friction varies with the speed of walking, providing a swing phase control that is responsive to the client's speed of gait.[15,17]

Extension aids are found in many mechanical knee joints. Generally, the aid is a spring built into the knee mechanism that enhances terminal knee extension at the end of swing phase.

Stance control mechanical knee mechanisms may be a manual lock knee or a weight activated mechanism (see Fig. 7.1). A brake is activated at heel contact and remains active throughout the stance phase. Some variability exists regarding how much weight is necessary to engage the mechanism and the range of knee flexion in which the brake will operate. Generally the mechanism operates within the first 20 degrees of knee flexion. If the knee is not fully extended as the client puts weight on the prosthesis, the knee will not buckle. These stance control knees are sometimes referred to as "safety" knees, a misnomer that may be misleading to the client. Unlike manual lock knees, stance phase control knees function as brakes rather than as locks.

The manual lock knee provides absolute stance phase control but does not swing as the knee remains locked in extension throughout the gait cycle. Manual lock knees have a locking mechanism that is activated by the client when standing and disengaged when ready to sit. They are occasionally used for individuals with bilateral amputations or those whose occupations may require considerable standing in one place.

Hydraulic Knee Mechanisms

Hydraulic knee mechanisms are similar to pneumatic systems except that the resistive medium is a silicone oil rather than air. The greater viscosity of the silicone oil increases the range of responses and is not subject to changes with extremes of temperatures. Hydraulic mechanisms provide a normal heel rise and forward swing appropriate to the client's speed of walking. Although hydraulic mechanisms are heavier than sliding friction units, they do not neces-

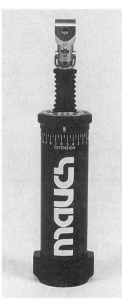

FIGURE 7.27
Heinski-Mauch Swing N Stance (S-N-S) hydraulic knee control system. (With permission from Mauch Laboratories, Inc.)

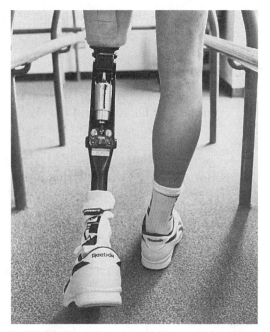

FIGURE 7.28
Endolite Intelligent Knee Control System. (With permission from the Endolite Corporation of North America.)

sarily feel heavier to the client because the more normal gait feel reduces energy expenditures.

Some hydraulic knee mechanisms provide swing phase and stance phase control. The Heinske Mauch Swing N Stance (S-N-S) (Mauch Laboratories Inc., Seattle, Washington) knee control system (Fig. 7.27), for example, is a sophisticated unit that allows separate adjustments for heel rise and terminal swing and provides a high degree of resistance to knee flexion when weight is borne on the prosthesis. The hyperextension moment at the knee that occurs as the individual rolls over the foot disengages the stance control mechanisms, allowing a smooth heel off and knee flexion for swing phase. The stance control mechanism allows some clients to walk downstairs step over step. The mechanism does not require voluntary hip extension for stance phase control; to the contrary, hip extension in stance releases the stance control mechanism allowing for unrestricted knee flexion. PTs and PTAs training clients fitted with the S-N-S are advised to obtain training information from their local prosthetist. The Endolite intelligent prosthesis (Endolite Corporation, Centerville, Ohio) incorporates a knee mechanism with a wide range of stance and swing phase control, a lightweight socket, and a multiflex ankle system designed to support a wide range of activities (Fig. 7.28).

Prostheses for Hip Disarticulation/Transpelvic Amputation

Hip disarticulations and transpelvic prostheses are similar in components and alignment. The only difference is the socket. Rejection rates for these prostheses are high as the gait cadence is slow and requires great energy. Wearers find the prostheses heavy and uncomfortable.[18–20]

SOCKETS

The hip disarticulation socket is made of plastic, encloses the ischial tuberosity for weight bearing, and covers the iliac crest for stability in swing phase (Fig. 7.29). It encircles the pelvis with an anterior slit to allow ease of donning and doffing. The medial aspect is cut to provide clearance for the other leg and genitalia. Relief is provided over the anterior and posterior iliac spines. Variations in socket construction include a lateral opening diagonal socket and a full socket similar to the transpelvic that encloses both iliac crests for stability.

The transpelvic socket is similarly made except that it must include the contralateral iliac crest for proper stabilization and suspension (see Fig. 7.29). Weight bearing is primarily on the remaining soft tissue and the contralateral ischium. Care must be taken when constructing both sockets so that no excess pressure exists on a bony prominence or in the perineum.

Both sockets can be made of rigid or flexible plastic and padded for increased comfort on weight bearing. Recently, flexible silicone rubber sockets in a rigid frame have been developed. The sockets provide a softer, more intimate fit that increases range of motion and comfort.[20]

HIP, KNEE, AND FOOT

The single axis unlocked hip joint is attached to the anterior aspect of the socket to provide stance phase stability and ease of swing phase. (See Chap. 8 for details of alignment.) A spring assisted mechanism may be incorporated for young, active clients to aid in initiating swing phase. Hip and knee motion is controlled by extension straps and alignment (Fig. 7.30).

Any knee joint can be used in the hip disarticulation prosthesis. The constant friction knee is probably used most often because of its light weight and lower cost. Any of the prosthetic feet discussed at the beginning of this chapter can be used with these prostheses.

Prostheses for Bilateral Amputations

BILATERAL TRANSTIBIAL AMPUTATIONS

The individual with two transtibial amputations uses the same components as an individual with one transtibial amputation. The person may require feet with somewhat softer heels for increased stance stability.

BILATERAL TRANSFEMORAL AMPUTATIONS

Ambulation with bilateral transfemoral prostheses is energy consuming, slow, and awkward. Most older individuals prefer to use a wheelchair rather than attempt ambulation.

Stubby prostheses or "stubbies" (see Chap. 5) are generally prescribed only for individuals who are motivated to ambulate but who are not candidates for fitting with full length prostheses. They may also be used as temporary pros-

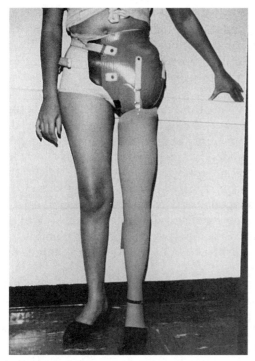

FIGURE 7.29
Endoskeletal hemipelvectomy prosthesis.

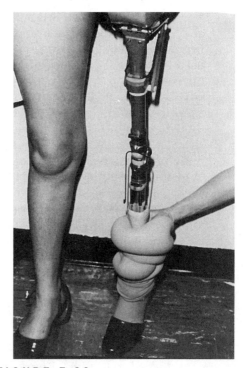

FIGURE 7.30
Endoskeletal components of the hemipelvectomy prosthesis. Note the elastic band posteriorly from socket to upper thigh in control swing phase.

theses. Stubbies are transfemoral prosthetic sockets set on rockers or prosthetic feet and are used to help the person move around in an upright position. Many people find stubbies cosmetically unacceptable because of the extreme reduction in height. Ambulation on stubbies obligates exaggerated trunk rotation. Short canes or crutches are usually needed for support. Sitting in a chair and climbing stairs are very difficult because of the shortness of the prostheses. The limbs also protrude in front of the chair while the person is sitting because they lack knee joints. If the wearer becomes proficient in walking with stubbies, then the question of whether to have full length prostheses can be raised. Although the person may be very stable when walking with stubbies, the lack of height is a likely source of embarrassment. Factors to be weighed when considering longer artificial limbs are the increased demands on the cardiovascular system, the decreased balance and stability caused by the elevated center of gravity, and the use of knee joints. If good balance, endurance, and motivation are present, then standard limbs may be considered.

Research and Development

New designs, materials, and fitting procedures are being developed and tested. Improved international communications have led to greater sharing of information, research, and technology.[21,22] Computer assisted design and computer assisted manufacture (CAD and CAM) systems are used more frequently. CAD and CAM systems allow faster fitting, construction, and delivery. Currently in limited use mainly for transtibial and transfemoral sockets, the system is being used increasingly in Veterans Administration hospitals and in other countries. Increased use of personal computers in local prosthetic facilities will also increase the practicality of such systems.

Flexible silicone sockets have allowed innovations in fitting not before thought possible. Transtibial suction sockets are becoming more common; the silicone soft socket has been used at the transfemoral and transpelvic levels. Early problems with the silicone suspension in the transfemoral prosthesis included intermittent loss of suction and some rotation between the liner and the socket. These problems have recently been reported as resolved; consequently, increased use of the silicone suction suspension with individuals of all ages is anticipated.[24] A shock absorbing gel liner has been developed for use with either transtibial or transfemoral sockets. Although this liner is thicker and heavier than the silicone liner, the intimate fit provides a snug and comfortable interface.

Considerable research is also being done on knee and ankle mechanisms. Some hydraulic knee mechanisms can now be computer adjusted to reflect minor changes in gait patterns and to provide some stance phase stability. Multiaxis systems allow knee flexion to 130 or 150 degrees. Turntables and torque mechanisms exist that allow the individual wearing a transfemoral limb to sit cross legged or to pivot around during a golf swing. A myoelectric knee mechanism is in development.

Multimovement ankle mechanisms functioning with dynamic response feet are being fabricated of lightweight yet durable materials, such as carbon fibers and plastics. There are lower extremity prostheses that allow clients to participate in most sports activities, including water sports, and wear shoes with varied height heels without changing feet or alignment.

A continuing problem in prosthetic wear is the lack of direct sensory feedback. Sabolich and Ortega[25] reported on initial work on a sensor incorporated into the foot to provide feedback to the residual limb. In an early study, the researchers reported that subjects increased prosthetic standing balance by 24 percent.

On the negative side, complex components are expensive and the extra charges are usually not reimbursed by third party payers. Government support of prosthetic research has also dwindled, increasing the cost of research and development and subsequent cost of components. Cost containment measures will probably affect the development of new, more complex, and more widely functional components. It behooves the therapist working with clients who have lost a limb to remain familiar with new developments to help educate the client regarding available components.

SUMMARY

The field of prosthetic components is rapidly changing. PTs and PTAs need to work closely with prosthetists in their local areas to help select the most functional components for each client. Much of the information gathered during the postsurgical period is helpful in component selection.

GLOSSARY

Alignment stability	Stance phase knee extension and stability created by aligning the knee joint posterior to the vertical knee axis line.
Components	The parts of a prosthesis.
Dynamic alignment	The slight movement of foot or knee component in relationship to the socket to provide the client with an optimum gait. This can only be done after the client has learned how to walk with the prosthesis.
Endoskeletal	A lightweight metal tube to connect the components. The shank is covered by a soft foam cover that matches the color and configuration of the other leg.
Exoskeletal	Wood or rigid polyurethane covered with rigid plastic lamination.
Myoelectric	The stimulation of muscle action by electric current.
Pistoning	The dropping of a prosthesis away from the residual limb during swing phase of gait. Usually occurs with inadequate suspension.
Residuum	Residual limb.
Shank	The part of a prosthesis corresponding to the lower leg of the unamputated limb, or the part that connects the foot to the socket (transtibial) or knee unit (transfemoral). The shank includes the pylon and cosmetic cover of the endoskeletal and is the finished part of the exoskeletal.
Socket	The component into which the residual limb is inserted.
Static alignment	The placement of the prosthetic components in proper relationship to each other in the standing position. The socket, knee component (if used), and foot are placed to duplicate the trochanter, knee, and ankle relationships of the nonamputated leg.
Voluntary knee control	Stance phase stability of the transfemoral prosthesis that is controlled by the client's extension of the residual limb against the posterior wall of the socket.

REFERENCES

1. Culham, ET, Peat, M, and Newell, E: Analysis of gait following below-knee amputation: A comparison of the SACH and single-axis foot. Physiotherapy Canada 36:237–242, 1984.
2. Brouwer, BJ, Allard, P, and Labelle, H: Running patterns of juveniles wearing SACH and single-axis foot components. Arch Phys Med Rehabil 70:128–134, 1989.
3. Winter, DA, and Sienko, SE: Biomechanics of below-knee amputee gait. J Biomech 21:361–367, 1988.
4. Campbell, JW, and Childs, CW: The S.A.F.E. foot. Orthot Prosthet 34:3–16, 1980.
5. Burgess, EM, Hittenberger, DA, Forsgren, SM, and Lindh, D: The Seattle prosthetic foot: A design for active sports: Preliminary studies. Journal of Prosthetic Orthotics, 37:25–31, 1983.

6. Kapp, S, and Cummings, D: Transtibial amputations: Prosthetic management. In Bowker, JH, and Michael, JW (eds.): Atlas of Limb Prosthetics: Surgical, Prosthetic, and Rehabilitation Principles, ed 2, Mosby-Year Book, St. Louis, 1992, pp. 453–478.

7. Czerniecki, JM, Munro, CF, and Gitter, A: A comparison of the power generation/absorption characteristics. Arch Phys Med Rehabil 68:636, 1987.

8. Czerniecki, JM, and Gitter, A: Impact of energy-storing prosthetic feet on below-knee amputation gait (abstract). Arch Phys Med Rehabil: 70(13):918, 1989.

9. Macfarlane, PA, Nielsen, DH, Shurr, DG, and Meier, K: Gait comparisons for below-knee amputees using a Flex-Foot versus a conventional prosthetic foot. Journal of Prosthetics and Orthotics 3:150–161, 1991.

10. Wirta, RW, Mason, R, Calvo, K, and Goldbranson, FL: Effect on gait using various prosthetic ankle-foot devices. J Rehabil Res Dev 28:13–24, 1991.

11. Childress, DS, and Knox, EH: Dynamic response prosthetic feet and their role in human ambulation. Paper presented at the 8th World Congress of the International Society for Prosthetic and Orthotics, Melbourne, Australia, April 1995 and published on the worldwide web.

12. Pritham, CH: Biomechanics and shape of the above-knee socket considered in light of the ischial containment concept. Prosthet Orthot Int 14:9–21, 1990.

13. Haberman, LJ, Bedotto, RA, and Colodney, EJ: Silicone-only suspension (SOS) for the above-knee amputee. Journal of Prosthetics and Orthotics 4:76–85, 1992.

14. Valenti, TG: Experiences with Endoflex: A monolithic thermoplastic prosthesis for below-knee amputees. Journal of Prosthetics and Orthotics 3:43–50, 1991.

15. Schuch, CM: Prosthetic management In Bowker, JH and Michael, JW (eds.): Atlas of Limb Prosthetics: Surgical, Prosthetic, and Rehabilitation Principles, ed 2. Mosby-Year Book, St. Louis, 1992, pp. 509–534.

16. Gottschalk, FA, Kourosh, S, Stills, M, et al: Does socket configuration influence the position of the femur in above-knee amputations? Journal of Prosthetics and Orthotics 2:94–102, 1990.

17. Mooney, V, and Quigley, MJ: Above-knee amputations: Section II, prosthetic management. In American Academy of Orthopedic Surgeons: Atlas of Limb Prosthetics, ed 2. St. Louis, Mosby-Year Book, 1981, pp. 384–401.

18. Jensen, JS, and Mandrup-Poulsen, T: Success rate of prosthetic fitting after major amputation of the lower limb. Prosthet Orthot Int 7:119–122, 1983.

19. Shurr, DG, Cook, TM, and Buckwalter, JA: Hip disarticulation: A prosthetic follow-up. Orthot Prosthet 37:50–57, 1983.

20. Van der Waarde, T, and Michael, JW: Prosthetic management. In Bowker, JH, and Michael, JW (eds.): Atlas of Limb Prosthetics: Surgical, Prosthetic, and Rehabilitation Principles, ed. 2. Mosby-Year Book, St. Louis, 1992, pp. 539–552.

21. Pritham, CH: Emerging trends in lower-limb prosthetics: Research and development. In Bowker, JH, and Michael, JW (eds.): Atlas of Limb Prosthetics: Surgical, Prosthetic, and Rehabilitation Principles, ed. 2. Mosby-Year Book, St. Louis, 1992, pp. 655–662.

22. Michael, JW, and Bowker, JH: Prosthetics/Orthotics research for the twenty-first century: Summary of 1992 conference proceedings. Journal of Prosthetics and Orthotics 6:100–107, 1994.

23. Steele, AL: A survey of clinical CAD/CAM use. Journal of Prosthetics and Orthotics. 6:42–47, 1994.

24. Haberman, LJ: Silicone-only suspension (SOS) with socket-loc and the ring for the lower limb. Journal of Prosthetics and Orthotics 7:2–14, 1995.

25. Sabolich, JA, and Ortega, GM: Sense of feel for lower-limb amputees: A phase-one study. Journal of Prosthetics and Orthotics 6:36–41, 1994.

chapter eight

Lower Extremity Prosthetic Management

OBJECTIVES

At the end of this chapter, all students are expected to:

1 Describe the factors that mitigate against prosthetic fitting.

2 Describe major gait deviations that may be exhibited by individuals walking with a transtibial or transfemoral prosthesis.

3 Describe the critical components of the prosthetic training program.

4 Compare and contrast the training program for clients with one or two transtibial prostheses.

In addition, physical therapy (PT) students are expected to:

1 Outline the steps in a transtibial and transfemoral prosthetic evaluation.

2 Establish functional goals for an individual with a transfemoral or transtibial prosthesis.

3 Design a prosthetic training program for an individual with a transfemoral or a transtibial prosthesis.

The first step in the prosthetic management of individuals with lower extremity amputations is to determine who is and is not a candidate for prosthetic fitting. The decision may be made by an amputee clinic team or an individual physician, or may be initiated by a PT. The PT or PT assistant (PTA) working in home health care or a rehabilitation center is in a particularly good position to make a referral to a local clinic or to discuss prosthetic fitting with the surgeon.

case studies

Each of our clients has been referred to the amputee clinic for prosthetic evaluation today. Prior to clinic, each person is evaluated by a physical therapist. The information is used by the clinic team in its decision making.

Diana Magnolia: It is now 12 weeks since her discharge from the hospital. Ms. Magnolia has been referred to the amputee clinic by the home health PT. Figure 8.1 shows the preclinic assessment for Ms. Magnolia.

Ha Lee Davis: It is now 8 weeks since his surgery. He is wearing his third plaster of Paris postsurgical socket. This socket has a foot and pylon attached that can be removed for inspection of the residual limb. He is referred by the outpatient physical therapist. Figure 8.2 is his preclinic assessment.

Benny Pearl: It is now 5 months since his discharge from the hospital. Following discharge he went to a rehabilitation center for 2 weeks, then went home. He has been referred to the amputee clinic by the vascular surgeon. Figure 8.3 is his preclinic assessment.

Subjective: "I sure would like a leg so I can walk"

Objective:

Active ROM Left Lower Extremity:
Knee Flexion/ Extension = 120–10 degrees
Hip Flexion/Extension = 120–10 degrees
Hip Abduction/Adduction and Rotation :WNL

Strength Left Lower Extremity:
Knee Flexion/Extension: G-(4-/5)
Hip: all musculature grossly Good to Good + range (4 to 4+/5)

Circumferential Measurement:	L	R
At tibial tubercle	13-3/4"	14"
1" below	13-1/8"	13-3/8"
2" below	12-7/8"	13-3/8"

Right Lower Extremity:
Toes are cool to touch, hairless with severe clubbing of toe nails. Client has small beginning ulceration just behind the heel which is being dressed by family and home health nurse. Decreased sensation to touch in right foot and ankle to malleoli, more pronounced on plantar surface of foot and over toes. Cannot consistently discern dull and sharp on plantar surface of foot and dorsum of toes. Can ambulate independently in the parallel bars and with a walker.

Home Health:
Therapist report confirms above measurements. Has been using the walker around the house and outside but complains of cramping in right lower extremity after about 50 feet. Client's teen age son has been helping her wrap the residual limb over the shrinker since the residual limb has decreased in size. She verbalizes a desire and need for a prosthesis. Social services have been contacted regarding obtaining proper shoes and an individually designed shoe insert for the right foot.

Assessment:
Ms. Magnolia has a well-healed non edematous residual limb, independent mobility skills and is ready for prosthetic fitting.

Plan:
Refer to clinic for prosthetic prescription.

FIGURE 8.1
Preclinic assessment for Diana Magnolia.

Subjective: I've gone back to school but I can't work; I hope I can get a real leg now.

Objective:
Residual limb length–18 cm; well healed, non sensitive, non edematous

Circumference:
@ Medial Tibial Plateau (MTP) level =31 cm; @ 5 cm = 33 cm; @ 10 cm = 33 cm; @ 18 cm = 32 cm
ROM and Muscle strength Right hip and knee within normal limits
Wearing 3rd temporary plaster of Paris removable post operative prosthesis.
Independent in all mobility activities with crutches and prosthesis.

Social Note:
Mr. Davis is finishing his last year of high school and is covered by private insurance. He was working part time in a fast food restaurant and did not have specific vocational or educational plans. He has been referred to the Department of Vocational Rehabilitation for evaluation.

Assessment:
Mr. Davis is ready for prosthetic fitting

Plan:
Refer to clinic for prosthetic prescription.

FIGURE 8.2
Preclinic assessment for Ha Lee Davis.

Betty Childs: Betty underwent a series of chemotherapy and radiation therapy treatments following surgery. She has now completed all adjuvant therapy and is referred to the amputee clinic at the request of the orthopedic surgeon who performed the amputation. It is 3 months since the amputation. Figure 8.4 is her preclinic assessment.

Subjective: "My stump just aches all over."

Objective:

Active ROM Right Hip:
Flexion/Extension: 130–10 degrees; Abduction: 25 degrees; adduction: 5 degrees.

Passive ROM Right Hip:
Flexion/Extension: 140–10;

Muscle Strength Right Hip:
Flexion: G+(4+/5); Extension: F (3/5) (measured sidelying; cannot get prone)

Circumference Residual Limb:
Residual limb is well healed but still slightly edematous with no change in measurements for the past 3 weeks. No specific areas of tenderness. Patient had some difficulty with wrapping and was fitted with transfemoral shrinker which he states he wears all the time.

Functional Status:
Mr. Pearl is independent in all wheelchair transfer activities; he generally uses a wheelchair at home except that he uses the walker to go to the bathroom. He is independent in all self care except for bathing as he cannot get into the bathtub. Mr. Pearl is able to ambulate independently in the parallel bars and can use a walker within the department with contact guard. Left lower extremity is hairless below the knee with evidence of dysvascularity in the foot. Client states it will swell when he sits all day; occasionally wears an elastic stocking on the leg. He complains of some night cramping. No evidence of ulcerations. Sensation appears present throughout and Mr. Pearl can differentiate sharp and dull on foot.

Assessment:
Somewhat obese individual who has the balance to ambulate with a walker but is limited by PVD of the (L) leg and decreased endurance. States a desire for a prosthesis but may not have a realistic awareness of the demands of transfemoral prosthetic ambulation.

Plan:
Refer to prosthetic clinic for further determination of whether to fit or not.

FIGURE 8.3
Preclinic assessment for Benny Pearl.

Subjective:
I'm glad that the chemotherapy is finished. It made me so weak.
Betty states she stopped wearing the AK shrinker in the past two weeks because she lost weight and it did not fit well.

Objective:
Residual limb well healed, conical, no edema.
Length from greater trochanter to end of limb = 32 cm
Circumference: At ischial level = 40 cm; 5 cm = 38 cm; 8 cm = 29 cm; 13 cm = 26 cm;
28 cm =26 cm.
Gross muscle strength Right hip is within normal limits;
Active ROM normal in all ranges except active and passive hip extension prone possible to about 5 degrees.
Independent on crutches in all ambulation and elevation activities.

Social Note:
Betty has returned to school this past week. She is financially covered by Crippled Children's Services. She and her family are anxious for her to get a prosthesis to return to normal life.

Assessment:
Betty has lost some weight which she may regain. She is ready for prosthetic fitting.

Plan:
Refer to prosthetic clinic for fitting with temporary transfemoral prosthesis.

FIGURE 8.4
Preclinic assessment for Betty Childs.

CASE STUDY ACTIVITY

Explore your beliefs about this statement. "Everyone is entitled to be fitted with a prosthesis." What conditions have to exist for a client not to be a prosthetic candidate? What does the research literature reflect on long term prosthetic use?

Prosthetic Fitting Decisions

No general rule can be safely applied to all clients when deciding whether or not to fit the person with a prosthesis. The client is part of the decision making process, but wanting a prosthesis is not sufficient. Many people are not aware of the physiological demands of prosthetic ambulation, particularly at transfemoral levels. The development of lightweight prostheses and stabilizing knee mechanisms has made it possible to fit more individuals successfully than in the past; however, some consideration for not fitting is necessary.

ENERGY EXPENDITURE

Individuals with transtibial amputations reach a higher level of function and use less energy for ambulation than individuals with transfemoral amputations.[1–3] Walking speed affects energy use; the faster one walks, the more energy is expended. Most individuals select a walking speed that maintains a comfortable level of oxygen consumption. Individuals with transtibial amputations are reported to expend significantly less energy when walking with a prosthesis at a self selected speed than when walking on crutches without a prosthesis; the difference in energy expenditure for individuals using a transfemoral prosthesis or walking on crutches, however, is not statistically significant.[4] Results of studies of energy expenditure between individuals using transtibial and transfemoral prostheses vary if walking speed is client selected or externally imposed. A comparison of a matched group of normal subjects and of people with unilateral transfemoral prostheses revealed no significant difference in oxygen consumption when the clients selected their own walking speed. People with transfemoral prostheses, however, walked at lower and less efficient speeds.[5] Most studies of energy expenditure indicate little difference in oxygen consumption between normal subjects and those with either a transtibial or transfemoral amputation, but do indicate a significant decrease in walking speed and walking efficiency with the higher level of amputation.[6] Individuals with unilateral transfemoral amputations are more likely to stop using the prosthesis than individuals with unilateral transtibial amputations. Associated medical problems such as coronary artery disease, hypertension, limited premorbid function and level of amputation have the most influence on long term outcomes.[7,8] The higher the level of the amputation, the heavier the prosthesis, and the greater number of artificial joints the person must control to achieve a smooth, energy efficient gait.

TRANSTIBIAL LEVEL AMPUTATIONS

Most individuals with transtibial amputations can be fitted with a prosthesis. Flexion contractures, scars, poorly shaped residual limbs, and adherent skin are not necessarily contraindications, even though such problems create difficulty with socket fit and prosthetic alignment. Circulatory problems in the non-amputated extremity, unless they are so severe as to preclude ambulation, are indications for fitting at the earliest possible time since bipedal ambulation reduces stress on the remaining extremity. Additionally, the individual who has learned to ambulate with one prosthesis is more likely to be able to ambulate with two. There are few contraindications to fitting someone with a transtibial amputation except contraindications to ambulation itself. Individuals who were not ambulatory before surgery for reasons other than the problems that necessitated the amputation will probably not be ambulatory afterwards. Individuals who were nonambulatory and debilitated because of infection, loss of diabetic control, and ulcers, however, may well regain the strength and coordination necessary for ambulation after the diseased limb has been removed. The increased energy requirements of ambulating with two prostheses may preclude fitting for individuals with cardiac disease and limited respiratory reserves. Generally, individuals requiring nursing or custodial care will not be able to use a prosthesis; often equipment sent to a nursing home becomes lost and fitting such individuals may be a waste of limited resources.

TRANSFEMORAL LEVEL AMPUTATIONS

Many people with a unilateral transfemoral amputation can become functional prosthetic users with or without external support. The physiological demands of walking with a transfemoral prosthesis are considerably higher than walking with a transtibial prosthesis, however, and not all individuals have the necessary balance, strength, and energy reserves. A transfemoral prosthesis is heavier than a transtibial prosthesis; control of the artificial knee joint requires considerable balance and coordination. Severe hip flexion contractures, weakness or paralysis of hip musculature, poor balance and coordination, or severe organic brain syndrome may mitigate against successful ambulation. The person's level of activity and participation in the preprosthetic program help to determine potential for prosthetic ambulation. The individual who is willing to learn to ambulate on the remaining extremity and shows the ability to expend the necessary energy to participate in an active preprosthetic program is a candidate for fitting. A person who is content to sit in a wheelchair except during scheduled therapy sessions, however, probably will not become a successful prosthetic user. A temporary prosthesis is a good assessment tool, although cost must be considered.

Most individuals with amputations at hip levels are young and learn to use a prosthesis relatively easily. Although early fitting is physically and psychologically beneficial, client involvement in chemotherapy or radiation therapy may delay fitting. Radiation therapy often burns the skin, making fitting impossible until the skin has healed. Clients undergoing chemotherapy often feel ill, lose weight, and do not have the stamina to participate in a prosthetic training program. The preprosthetic program is individually adjusted and supportive until chemotherapy is complete. If the person has lost considerable weight, fitting will have to be delayed since it is difficult to adjust a prosthesis for the eventual increase in weight.

BILATERAL AMPUTATIONS

The decision to fit or not fit a person with bilateral amputations is difficult. Young, agile individuals are generally good candidates for prosthetic fitting. Most people with bilateral transtibial amputations can become functional with prostheses. Essentially, the same criteria are applied as for a client with one amputation, although greater energy expenditure is necessary for ambulation with two transtibial prostheses. Individuals with bilateral transtibial amputations reach a higher level of independent function than individuals with one transfemoral and one transtibial amputation or those with bilateral transfemoral amputations.[3,9,10]

Ambulation with one transfemoral and one transtibial prosthesis requires considerably more energy than ambulation with bilateral transtibial prostheses. Individuals with transfemoral and transtibial amputations have a better chance of becoming ambulatory if the first amputation was at the transfemoral level, and if the person successfully used a transfemoral prosthesis before losing the other leg. Most older individuals with two transfemoral amputations do not become successful prosthetic wearers because of the energy and balance requirements. The person who has lost both extremities needs more strength, better coordination, better balance, and greater cardiorespiratory reserves than the person who has lost one. The decision to fit or not to fit is made after careful individual evaluation of the person's total potential and needs.

FACTORS AFFECTING PROSTHETIC WEAR

Residual limb problems delay prosthetic rehabilitation. Skin problems such as dermatitis, furuncles, cysts, and infections usually require careful skin hygiene, occasional medication, and avoidance of the prosthesis. Soap residue left on the skin can be irritating; the client must be taught to rinse the residual limb, socks, and socket thoroughly after washing.

Clients with vascular disease must watch for excessive pressure on the residual limb from the prosthetic socket. Necrosis of distal tissue can occur even after wound healing. Individuals with diabetes who may have decreased sensation need to learn to inspect the residual limb carefully after each wearing to note any areas of redness or pressure. If any skin around the incision adheres to the distal end of the bone, the forces created by prosthetic wear may cause pain or abrasions. Care must be taken during healing to prevent adhesions by careful massage and movement of the skin around the bone. Occasionally bone spurs develop, causing excessive pressure on the overlying skin. Children are subject to problems created by bone growth through the skin at the end of the residual limb (see Chap. 11).

Some clients develop a painful residual limb that interferes with the ability to wear a prosthesis. Pain may be of physiological or psychogenic origin and often encompasses elements of both. Chronic pain is difficult to treat. A painful phantom limb can be extremely resistant to treatment, as discussed in Chapter 5. A neuroma is a natural sequela of the transection of a nerve. The size and location of the neuroma are critical; a small neuroma located in soft tissue well above the distal end of the residual limb will usually not interfere with prosthetic wear. Large superficial neuromas may be compressed between the socket wall and the bone, causing pain. Relieving the socket wall at the site of the neuroma may resolve the problem. Injecting the neuroma with an analgesic or steroid formula may be necessary, but, since the relief is only temporary, the injection may need to be repeated several times. In more stubborn instances, surgery to excise the neuroma may be indicated. Centrocentral anastomosis or inserting a nerve graft at the neuroma in an end to end connection has been reported to eliminate neuroma pain in a small sample of clients.[11] The use of ice or electrotherapy has sometimes been successful and should be tried first.

Pain during or after wearing the prosthesis may be caused by a problem with the prosthetic socket. Minor impingement of the socket in areas of superficial tendons or excessive soft tissue may only cause problems after prolonged wearing. Careful inspection of the stump/socket interface is necessary to make sure that the pain is not due to changes in socket pressure, excessive socket pressure in one area, edema, or changes in the client's weight.

The Prosthetic Evaluation

The first step in prosthetic management is to make sure that the prosthesis fits properly and that it is as prescribed by the clinic team. Figures 8.5 and 8.6 reproduce forms used to evaluate prostheses. If the client is a new prosthetic wearer, only the initial parts of the evaluation are performed; evaluation of gait is delayed until the person has learned to walk with a consistent gait pattern. Gait deviations are explored later in this chapter.

The evaluation is designed to ensure that the prosthesis fits appropriately, and that the wearer has adequate stability, and is satisfied with the device. In many clinics, the prosthetist initially delivers the appliance on the alignment instrument. Beginning evaluation and training are performed while the prosthesis is easily adjustable. It takes time for the client and the residual limb to adjust to the prosthesis. After optimal alignment and fit have been obtained, the prosthesis can be finished. Although alignment changes are easier with endoskeletal limbs, it is a good practice to have the prosthesis unfinished initially. When the prosthesis is delivered directly to the client without review by a clinic team, the prosthetist may finish the limb and alignment changes may be diffi-

Check Prosthesis Before Donning:
1. Is the prosthesis as prescribed?

Sitting:
2. Is the amputee comfortable while sitting with the sole of the shoe flat on the floor?
3. Is flaring of the posterior trim line adequate to accommodate the hamstring tendons?
4. Are the tissue rolls in the popliteal area excessive?
5. Is the residual limb forced out of the socket excessively?
6. Does the cuff suspension tend to loosen when the amputee sits?
7. Are the knees level?
8. Are the color and contour of the prosthesis similar to those of the sound leg?

Standing:
9. Does the client have any pain or discomfort?
10. Is the knee stable? Does the client have to resist to prevent the knee from being forced into flexion or extension?
11. Is the pelvis level when the amputee bears weight equally on both feet?
12. Is the pylon vertical?
13. Does the sole of the shoe maintain even contact with the floor?
14. Are tissue rolls around the trim line of the socket or of the cuff suspension minimal?
15. Is there gapping at the brim of the socket?
16. Is the residual limb in contact with the distal end of the socket?
17. Does the suspension cuff fit snugly over the superior patellar area?
18. Does the suspension cuff maintain its position as the amputee lifts the foot off the floor?

Walking:
19. Is the gait satisfactory?
   If the gait is not satisfactory, check the deviations.
   - Ball of foot more than 2.5 cm from the floor
   - Knee extended
   - Unequal stride length

   From heel strike to foot flat
   - Knee flexes jerkily
   - Maintains knee extension
   - Knee flexes abruptly

   At midstance
   - Lateral trunk bending exceeds 5 cm
   - Lateral displacement of socket exceeds 1.3 cm
   - Shoe not flat on the floor
   - No lateral or medial socket displacement

   Midstance to heel rise
   - Drop off
   - Prosthesis drops away from stance
   - Knee flexes jerkily

   At heel rise
   - Knee goes into extension

   During swing phase
   - Vaulting
   - Circumduction
   - Toe drags on floor

Check with Prosthesis Off:
20. Are there sock impressions over the entire residual limb?
21. Is the skin free of any abrasions, blisters, or excessive redness?
22. Is there any discoloration or discomfort?

FIGURE 8.5
Transtibial prosthetic checkout.

Check Prosthesis Before Donning:
1. Is the inside of the socket smoothly finished?
2. Does the socket meet socket specification (i.e., ischial containment or quadrilateral)?
3. Do all joints move freely and smoothly?
Comments on items 1–3: _____

Sitting:
4. Is the socket securely placed on the residual limb?
5. Does the length of the shin and thigh correspond to that of the shin and thigh of the unamputated leg?
6. Can the client sit comfortably without burning or pinching?
7. Is the client able to lean forward and reach her or his shoes?
Comments on items 4–7: _____

Standing:
8. Does the socket fit properly and comfortably?
9. Is the knee stable when weight is placed on the prosthesis?
10. Is the pelvis level when weight is borne evenly on both legs?
11. Is the client bearing weight properly for the type of socket?
12. Does the socket maintain good contact with the residual limb on all sides as the client shifts weight?
13. Is there an adductor roll?
14. Is there pressure on the pubic ramus?
Comments on items 9–14: _____

Walking:
15. Is suspension maintained during swing phase?
16. Is the socket stable against the lateral shift of the residual limb?
17. Is there optimum swing phase control?
18. Is level walking free of gait deviations? If not, check off the deviation observed on the following list:

   Heel contact to foot flat:
    ☐ Forceful heel strike
    ☐ Excessive external rotation of prosthesis
    ☐ Knee instability

   Midstance:
    ☐ Lateral trunk bending toward prosthesis side
    ☐ Lateral gapping of socket
    ☐ Abducted gait
    ☐ Lateral trunk bending toward prosthesis side
    ☐ Lateral gapping of socket
    ☐ Abducted gait

   Midstance to toe off:
    ☐ Premature heel rise
    ☐ Drop off
    ☐ Excessive lumbar lordosis
    ☐ Pelvic rise (climbing a hill)
    ☐ Delayed swing

   Swing phase:
    ☐ Cirumducted gait
    ☐ Lateral heel whip
    ☐ Terminal swing impact
    ☐ Excessive heel rise
    ☐ Medial heel whip
    ☐ Lack of knee flexion

Comments on gait _____
_____

After Ambulation:
19. Can prosthesis be removed easily?
20. Is residual limb free of any abrasions or areas of inflammation?

FIGURE 8.6
Transfemoral prosthetic checkout.

cult, particularly with exoskeletal limbs. Whenever possible, the therapist needs to ensure that initial evaluation and training are performed while the limb is still unfinished. Although the prosthetist performs a static and dynamic alignment before delivering the prosthesis, evaluation is the therapist's responsibility.

CASE STUDY ACTIVITY

Individually or in groups, review each item in the transfemoral and transtibial evaluation forms, preferably with a prosthesis. Explain the importance of each item and the effect on the client if the item does not meet standards. Be as specific as you can; pain is not an adequate answer. State *where* the pain will be felt and *how* it will affect function.

Transtibial Evaluation

Before any gait training can be instituted, the fit of the prosthesis must be evaluated. Areas to be evaluated include socket fit, suspension, comfort, leg length, and static alignment (Fig. 8.7). Table 8.1 depicts the key items of evaluation in the transtibial prosthesis and possible problems that may occur with misalignment. Contemporary fabrication methods reduce static alignment problems. It is critical, however, to check for socket comfort, initial socket flexion, total contact, and proper height before initiating gait training. If the prosthesis is

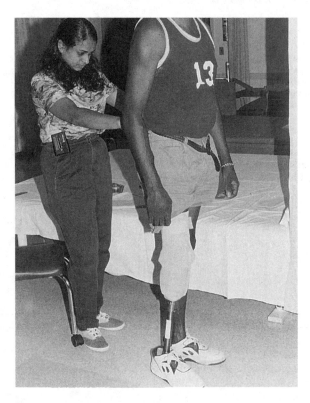

FIGURE 8.7
Checking the length of the prosthesis by checking for a level pelvis.

T A B L E 8 . 1 **STATIC TRANSTIBIAL PROSTHETIC EVALUATION**

Checkout Item	What to Check	Possible Problem
Sitting		
Is the amputee comfortable while sitting with the sole of the shoe flat on the floor?	Check for excessive pressure between stump and socket.	Excessive pressure can lead to skin abrasions.
Is there adequate flaring of the posterior trim line to accommodate the hamstring tendons?	Check for pressure on the hamstrings when sitting.	Client will keep leg outstretched when sitting to reduce pressure.
Are the tissue rolls in the popliteal area excessive?	Check the posterior wall of the socket.	Too much tissue may indicate inadequate anteroposterior dimensions.
Is the stump forced out of the socket excessively?	The stump rises out of the socket a little when sitting.	May indicate a socket that is too small or that the client is wearing too many socks.
Does the cuff suspension tend to loosen when the amputee sits?	The cuff suspension should loosen slightly when sitting.	Too tight or loose a cuff will lead to inadequate suspension.
Are the knees level?	The length of the shank should correspond to the other side.	May lead to gait deviations.
Are the color and contour of the prosthesis similar to those of the sound leg?	The finished prosthesis should match the other leg.	Poor cosmesis may lead to the client not wearing the prosthesis.
Standing		
Is the client comfortable?	Check stump/socket interface, particularly bony prominances.	Excessive pressures can lead to skin problems.
Is the knee stable? Does the client have to resist to prevent the knee from being forced into flexion or extension?	PTB socket aligned in 5 to 8 degrees of flexion.	Too much flexion will lead to counter knee extension and anterior distal pressure. Too little flexion can lead to end bearing.
Is the pelvis level when the amputee bears weight equally on both feet?	Palpate the iliac crests with client standing evenly on both feet.	A long or short prosthesis will lead to gait deviations.
Is the pylon vertical?	On weight bearing, check the pylon connecting the socket and foot.	See medial and lateral leaning pylons on gait deviations.
Does the sole of the shoe maintain even contact with the floor?	Check that the foot is fully on the floor on weight bearing.	May lead to excessive knee pressures on gait.
Are tissue rolls around the trim line of the socket or the cuff suspension minimal?	Check the edges of the stump at the socket line.	Excessive rolls may indicate a socket that is too tight proximally.
Is there gapping at the brim of the socket?	Check the edges of the stump at the socket line.	Gapping may indicate a socket that is too large proximally.
Is the residual limb in contact with the distal end of the socket?	Put a little ball of soft modeling clay at the end of the socket, then have the client bear weight. The displacement of the modeling clay indicates the extent of total contact.	Too little contact can cause distal end skin problems and a stretching pain. Too much can cause excessive pressure at the end of the stump and pressure pain.

Table continued on following page

T A B L E   8 . 1   **STATIC TRANSTIBIAL PROSTHETIC EVALUATION** (Continued)

Checkout Item	What to Check	Possible Problem
Does the suspension cuff fit snugly over the superior patellar area?	Check that the cuff is over the patella and not impinging on the patella.	Improper placement can interfere with proper suspension.
Does the suspension cuff maintain its position as the amputee lifts the foot off the floor?	On weight bearing, make a small pencil mark at the anterior socket brim. As the client lifts the leg with knee straight, the socket should not drop more than $\frac{1}{4}$ inch.	A loose prosthesis can cause skin abrasions and can lead to toe drag on swing phase.

uncomfortable, the client will not be able to learn a smooth, step over step gait. Pressure areas may also cause skin breakdowns that can jeopardize the status of the residual limb.

THE KNEE IN NORMAL GAIT

In each cycle of normal gait, the knee flexes and extends twice. Just before heel contact, the knee is extended or nearly so; it flexes to about 15 degrees at midstance, extending back to neutral or 5 degrees of flexion by terminal stance. The knee flexes again in early swing, then extends in terminal swing before the next heel contact. From heel contact to midstance, the quadriceps are active to decrease and control knee flexion while the hamstring muscles are quiet. Quadriceps action reaches its peak about midstance. Knee flexion in swing results mostly from momentum; the hamstring's function is mainly to decelerate hip flexion and to prevent knee hyperextension in terminal swing.[12]

SOCKET EVALUATION

The patellar tendon bearing (PTB) socket is aligned in 5 to 8 degrees of knee flexion to allow for better weight bearing on the patella tendon and to stimulate normal gait. Excessive socket flexion creates knee instability; the client extends the knee to counteract the instability and drives the anterior distal end of the tibia that is close to the skin against the wall of the socket causing pain and possible abrasion (Fig. 8.8). Insufficient socket flexion reduces the weight-bearing potential of the patellar tendon and medial tibial flares, causing the residual limb to press too hard on the bottom of the socket. Insufficient socket flexion can also decrease the effectiveness of quadriceps motion.

Total contact provides good kinesthetic feedback during ambulation and enhances venous return at the distal end of the residual limb. A space left between the end of the residuum and the socket may cause the skin to become callused and rough. Lack of total contact can also lead to distal edema.

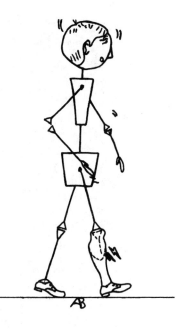

FIGURE 8.8
Heel contact to foot flat: extension force on knee creating anterior distal pressure. (Artist: Angie Britt)

The prosthesis must be held firmly on the residual limb by the suspension mechanism. Proper suspension is checked with the client standing. If the client is wearing something other than a sleeve suspension, a light pencil mark is made on the sock at the level of the anterior brim. The client is then asked to lift the prosthesis straight off the ground without bending the knee. The prosthesis should not drop more than about 1 centimeter. If the client is wearing a sleeve suspension, the therapist can place a finger at the anterior brim and have the client perform the same movement (Fig. 8.9). Any drop can be palpated.

The foot should be flat on the floor with body weight evenly distributed between the heel and toe of the prosthetic foot when the client is standing erect with weight placed equally on both feet. If the prosthesis is on the alignment instrument, the pylon connecting the foot to the socket should be perpendicular to the floor when the feet are a comfortable distance apart. The pylon will not be perpendicular if the client is bearing more weight on the nonamputated leg.

Transtibial Gait Analysis

NORMAL PROSTHETIC GAIT

Gait analysis is best done when viewing the client walking both from an anterior/posterior (AP) and a lateral (prosthetic side) point of reference. The therapist needs to obtain an overall impression of the gait, then focus on each part of the body individually to ensure a thorough analysis.

The client with a transtibial amputation walking with a well fitting and well aligned prosthesis exhibits a smooth, step over step pattern, with little trunk sway and with symmetrical arm movements. The gait requires minimum energy.

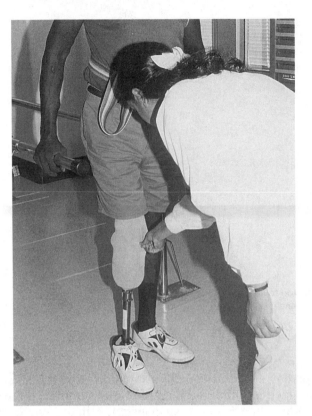

FIGURE 8.9
Checking for pistoning with sleeve suspension.

Heel Contact, Lateral View

The knee is slightly flexed, with the ball of the prosthetic foot no more than 4 centimeters from the floor. The pelvis and trunk are erect with the body weight being transferred from the nonamputated to the prosthetic leg.

Heel Contact to Foot Flat, Lateral View

Progressing toward foot flat, the knee flexes smoothly 10 to 15 degrees as the foot comes gently to the floor. The heel of the prosthetic foot compresses about 1.5 to 2 centimeters, depending on the person's weight and type of foot. The trunk remains balanced over the point of support.

Midstance, Anterior/Posterior View

At midstance, the client bears full weight on the prosthesis. The pelvis and upper body remain balanced over the prosthesis with no more than 2.5 centimeters of head or trunk sway toward the prosthetic side. The overall gait base is no more than 5 centimeters wide. There is minimum lateral socket displacement. On the alignment instrument, the pylon is perpendicular to the floor. The foot is flat on the floor.

Midstance, Lateral View

The prosthetic foot is flat on the floor, the knee is flexed 10 to 15 degrees and stable.

Midstance to Toe Off, Lateral and Anterior/Posterior Views

Weight progresses smoothly from the amputated to the nonamputated side with little head, trunk, or pelvic sway or drop. The knee flexes smoothly and there is no more than 5 centimeters between the two feet.

Swing Phase, Lateral View

The knee flexes easily and allows the toe to clear the floor. The socket remains securely on the residual limb. Step length is the same on each side.

Swing Phase, Anterior/Posterior View

The shank and foot swing in the line of progression and the pelvis remains level.

TRANSTIBIAL GAIT DEVIATIONS

Gait deviations may result from an improperly fitting socket, malaligned prosthesis, painful residual limb, or poor walking habits. Gait deviations increase energy consumption, can cause discomfort in the residual limb, and will limit functional use of the prosthesis. Identifying gait deviations early allows problems to be remedied before they become permanent. A client wearing a prosthesis with other than a sleeve suspension may exhibit a slight lateral thrust of the proximal brim of the socket during midstance. This movement results from the adduction of the femur and the slight valgus position of the normal knee. Normal floor reaction forces create a slight varus movement of the knee at midstance. As long as the movement is slight and does not affect comfort or stability, it is considered normal. Lateral thrust is usually not seen in individuals using a sleeve suspension unless the residual limb is very short. It is also not seen with individuals wearing closed patellar tendon supracondylar suprapatellar (PTSCSP) prostheses.

Heel Contact to Foot Flat

Excessive knee extension In the normal gait pattern, the knee flexes smoothly 10 to 15 degrees from heel contact to midstance. Flexion reduces the excursion of the body's center of gravity, allows absorption of the floor reaction forces generated at heel strike through the joints of the lower limb, and reduces the amount of energy required in gait. Keeping the knee extended increases the energy expended in walking; the deviation can best be seen from the side, observing the prosthetic knee from weight acceptance to midstance (see Fig. 8.8). The client reports a sense of walking uphill. Maintaining an extended knee with a socket aligned in flexion may lead to anterior distal pain and skin abrasion.

Extension also increases pelvic displacement; it may look as if the prosthesis is too long.

The two major prosthetic problems are a heel cushion that is too soft and a toe lever arm that is too long. The two deviations can be differentiated by watching the heel from heel contact to midstance. Knee extension may also result from inadequate gait training or weakness of the quadriceps.

1   **Heel cushion too soft.** A heel wedge that is too soft allows too rapid plantar flexion of the prosthetic foot. This premature contact of the foot with the floor tends to keep the knee in extension rather than allowing normal rolling over the foot.

2   **Too long toe lever arm (posterior displacement of the socket over the foot).** Posterior displacement of the socket brings the center of gravity line posteriorly, thereby increasing the length of the anterior segment or toe lever arm (Fig. 8.10). If the foot is set too far anteriorly under the socket, the length of the toe lever arm is increased and that of the heel lever arm is decreased. As the client progresses from heel contact to foot flat, the center of gravity moves anterior to the axis of rotation of the knee very quickly, thus forcing the knee into hyperextension. The client feels as if he or she is walking uphill as the length of the anterior support component increases.

Other possible causes of excessive knee extension include:

1   **Excessive plantar flexion of the foot** (Shoe with a lower heel). In normal walking, contact of the sole of the foot with the floor coincides approximately with the end of knee flexion and the beginning of knee extension. If the prosthetic foot is in an attitude of plantar flexion, foot flat occurs prematurely, preventing normal knee flexion after heel strike.

2   **Weakness of the quadriceps.** If the quadriceps are not strong enough to control the knee at heel strike, the client may compensate in much the same way as with anterodistal discomfort. These gait maneuvers tend to force the knee into extension and thereby lessen or eliminate the need for quadriceps activity.

3   **Habit.** Individuals who have established a pattern of walking with the knee held in extension after heel strike may continue to walk in the same manner when they are making the transition to a new transtibial prosthesis. Usually a brief period of instruction with early follow up suffices to establish a satisfactory walking pattern.

Knee Instability   Stability of the knee is critical to a smooth, energy efficient gait. A client who does not feel stable and fears that the knee may buckle will

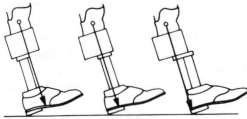

POSTERIOR SOCKET DISPLACEMENT

FIGURE 8.10
An overlong toe lever arm is caused by placement of the socket too far posterior on the foot. The first placement is correct. The other two are different degrees of incorrect.

not trust the limb. Depending on the cause, knee instability can be seen at initial or terminal stance (Fig. 8.11). The two common causes of prosthetic knee instability are a too short toe lever arm and a too hard heel cushion.

1   **Toe lever arm too short.** This problem is discussed in the section on terminal stance (pp. 158–159).
2   **Heel cushion too hard (dorsiflexed foot, higher heel shoe).** The compressibility of the prosthetic foot depends on the size, weight and activity level of the client. If the heel cushion is too hard, plantar flexion and shock absorption are insufficient, and the knee on the prosthetic side is forced into excessive flexion from heel contact to midstance. Knee instability and buckling may result. The client may try to maintain stability by extending the knee against the flexing forces, creating excessive pressure at the anterior distal end of the residual limb and possibly at the posterior proximal brim of the socket.

Excessive anterior distal pressure can lead to abrasions and skin breakdowns, because the distal end of the tibia is quite close to the socket wall.

Midstance

Excessive Raising or Dropping of the Hip on the Prosthetic Side

1   **Prosthesis too long.** If the prosthetic leg is longer than the unamputated leg, the client will raise the center of gravity over the support joint during stance phase. The deviation can best be seen from the rear by watching the prosthetic hip and shoulder during midstance. The client may also have difficulty bringing the prosthetic leg forward in swing and either bends the knee excessively or raises the body up on the toe of the sound leg to allow room to clear the prosthetic foot. The latter deviation is called **vaulting.**
2   **Prosthesis too short.** If the prosthetic leg is shorter than the unamputated leg, the person seems to be walking in a hole on the prosthetic side. The hip and shoulder on the amputated side drop at the beginning of stance phase (Fig. 8.12). This deviation can best be observed from the rear by watching the hip and shoulder at midstance. Some individuals prefer the prosthetic leg to be just slightly shorter than the sound leg, especially those who have had a lifelong discrepancy in leg lengths. Although ideally both legs should be the same length, comfort and function must be the guide in determining appropriate length alignment. This deviation is sometimes confused with "drop off," which occurs at terminal stance. In drop off, the prosthetic knee may have a tendency to buckle that usually does not occur with a prosthesis that is too short.

Wide Based Gait

If the base of support is moved laterally, support is lost medially during single foot stance. The client attempts to move the pelvis laterally to reach the support, exhibiting a wide based gait with the hips and the shoulders dropping laterally during stance phase (Fig. 8.13). Excess pressure is felt at the proximal lateral brim of the socket and the medial distal end of the residual limb. Two prosthetic problems are an outset foot and a medial leaning pylon. Both deviations can best be seen in either front or rear view; noting particularly movements of the trunk and shoulders in stance. The outset foot can be differentiated from the

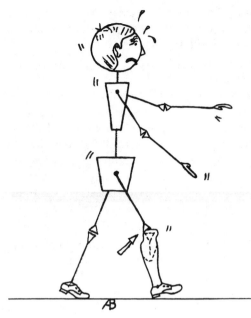

FIGURE 8.11
Heel contact to foot flat: knee instability. (Artist: Angie Britt)

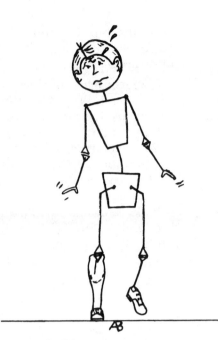

FIGURE 8.12
Midstance: prosthesis too short. (Artist: Angie Britt)

medial leaning pylon by looking at the pylon at midstance. The gait deviation may sometimes be noted if the person does not shift the weight properly over the prosthesis on stance. This training problem can be differentiated from a prosthetic problem by looking at the pylon at midstance and noting the width of the gait base.

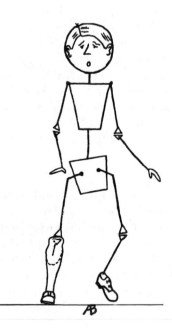

FIGURE 8.13
Midstance: wide based gait. (Artist: Angie Britt)

1 **Outset foot.** Normally, the foot is usually set 1 centimeter medial to a line from the center of the posterior wall to the floor. If the foot is set too far lateral to the line, the client loses support medially during stance. The sole of the shoe usually remains flat on the floor when the foot is outset.

2 **Medial leaning pylon.** Proper dynamic alignment places the pylon perpendicular at midstance. If the top of the pylon is medial to the bottom, the pylon is said to lean medially (Fig. 8.14). The client exhibits a wide based gait and seems to lose support medially as with an outset foot, but if the problem is a medial leaning pylon, the foot has more pressure on the medial side.

Narrow Based Gait and Excessive Lateral Thrust of the Prosthesis

A narrow based gait and thrust of the prosthesis laterally away from the knee at midstance often occur together and derive from the tendency of the prosthesis to rotate around the residual limb (Fig. 8.15). If the base of support (the prosthetic foot) is moved medially, support is lost laterally during single foot stance. Because there is no support for the pelvis in its normal alignment, it drops. In an attempt to maintain the pelvis level, the client may overcompensate and lean away from the prosthetic side on stance or may allow the drop to take place and lean laterally over the prosthesis on stance. In both instances, there is excess movement of the pelvis and shoulder either toward or away from the prosthesis. This gait deviation simulates a weak gluteus medius gait. The client reports increased pressure at the medial proximal and lateral distal ends of the socket. The socket may be seen to move laterally at midstance, opening a gap between the residual limb and the top of the socket. A slight lateral thrust of the knee on stance is considered normal; excessive lateral thrust can injure the knee joint.

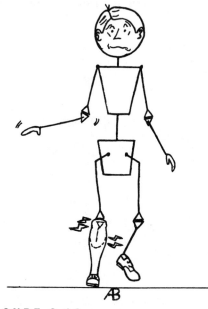

FIGURE 8.14

Midstance: medial leaning pylon results in excessive pressure on the proximal lateral and distal medial areas of the residual limb. (Artist: Angie Britt)

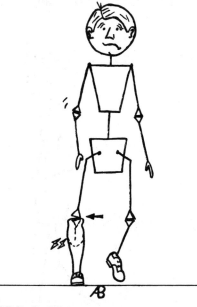

FIGURE 8.15

Midstance: lateral leaning pylon results in excessive pressure on the proximal medial and distal lateral areas of the residual limb. (Artist: Angie Britt)

Two common prosthetic causes are an excessively inset foot and a lateral leaning pylon. Both deviations can best be seen from the rear. In all deviations involving the alignment of the pylon, it is important to note the position at midstance and not at any other part of the gait cycle.

1   **Improper mediolateral tilt of the socket (lateral leaning pylon).** If the socket is set in abduction and the top of the pylon is more lateral than the bottom at midstance, the pylon is said to lean laterally (see Fig. 8.5). This increases pressure at the medial brim. In addition, the prosthetic foot is not flat on the floor and the weight is borne on the lateral border of the foot. These circumstances can be remedied by adducting the socket.

2   **Inset foot.** An inset foot results when the prosthetic foot is placed too far medial to the dynamic alignment line. At midstance, the sound extremity swings through the air so that all body weight is supported only by the prosthetic foot on the floor. If this supporting foot is too far medial to the line of action of forces transmitted through the socket, a force couple is created that tends to rotate the socket around the stump. In almost all instances, this lateral thrust can be minimized or eliminated by "out setting" the prosthetic foot slightly.

Terminal Stance

Knee Instability
Toe Lever Arm Too Short (Drop Off).   The toe lever arm provides support from midstance to terminal stance and allows the client to roll over the foot in a smooth manner. The heel lever arm provides support from heel strike to midstance allowing smooth descent of the prosthetic foot and controlled knee flexion. Just before heel off during normal gait, the knee is extending. At heel off or immediately thereafter, knee flexion begins. This change from extension to

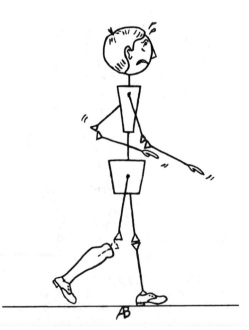

FIGURE 8.16
Terminal stance: drop off. (Artist: Angie Britt)

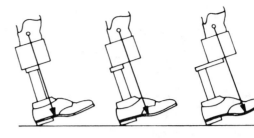

FIGURE 8.17
Too short a toe lever arm is caused by placement of the socket too far forward on the foot. The first placement is correct. The other two are different degrees of incorrect.

flexion coincides with the passing of the center of gravity over the metatarsophalangeal joints. If the body weight is carried over the metatarsophalangeal joints too soon, the resulting lack of anterior support allows premature knee flexion or drop off (Fig. 8.16). If the foot is placed too far posterior under the socket, the toe lever arm will be shortened and the client will not be supported in the terminal stance phase (Fig. 8.17). This premature loss of support causes the prosthetic knee to flex and the hip to drop sharply just before the end of stance. This deviation is called "drop off." It can best be seen from the lateral viewpoint by watching the hip and knee in terminal stance.

Knee Extension Vaulting
Toe Lever Arm Too Long. If the body weight is carried forward over a long toe lever arm, the knee joint remains in extension during the latter part of the stance phase and the client complains of a "walking uphill" sensation because the center of gravity is carried up and over the extended knee (Fig. 8.18). This prosthetic problem may be best viewed laterally.

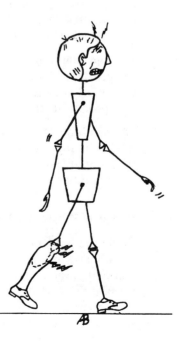

FIGURE 8.18
Terminal stance: too long a toe lever arm causes an extension moment. (Artist: Angie Britt)

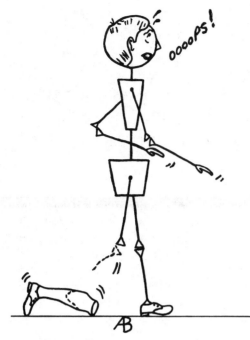

FIGURE 8.19
Swing phase: loss of suspension. (Artist: Angie Britt)

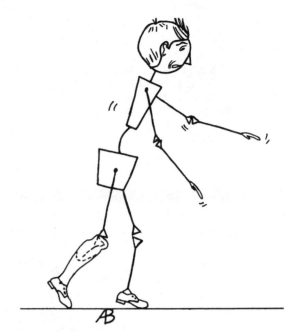

FIGURE 8.20
Swing phase: loss of suspension causes stubbing of the toe on the floor. (Artist: Angie Britt)

Swing Phase

Pistoning (Loss of Suspension) If the suspension mechanism is loose or inadequate, the prosthesis will slip as the foot leaves the ground for swing phase (Fig. 8.19). The toe of the prosthesis may catch on the ground or the movement of the socket against the skin may cause abrasions (Fig. 8.20).

Uneven Step Length Clients may develop the habit of taking a long step with the prosthesis and a short step with the unamputated leg. This may be the result of a poorly fitting socket causing pain, fear of putting weight on the prosthesis, or a prosthesis that is too long.

Circumduction Described as a semicircular swing of the prosthesis to the side during swing phase (Fig. 8.21), circumduction may be seen if the prosthesis is too long, the suspension is inadequate, or the person has difficulty flexing the hip and knee.

Transfemoral Prosthetic Evaluation

Table 8.2 lists the key items to check initially when evaluating a transfemoral prosthesis. In addition to the socket fit, suspension, comfort, leg length, and static alignment that is similar to the transtibial level, knee stability is an important consideration in the transfemoral limb. Two parts of knee control are alignment (involuntary control) and active hip extension (voluntary control). In most instances, the knee is placed in a line or slightly posterior to a line

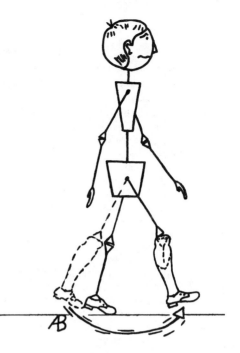

FIGURE 8.21
Swing phase: circumduction of the prosthesis.
(Artist: Angie Britt)

drawn from the trochanter to the ankle axis (**TKA line**) (Fig. 8.22). This allows the body weight line to fall anterior to the knee to create an extension moment on weight bearing. If the knee axis is on or anterior to the line, the body weight falls behind the knee creating flexion or an unstable moment. In the prosthesis fitted with a mechanical knee joint, the client extends the residual limb against the posterior wall of the prosthesis to maintain the knee in extension from heel strike to midstance. Setting the socket in about 5 degrees of flexion increases the client's ability to extend the hip without arching the back excessively. In clients with a hip flexion contracture, the socket must be set in 5 degrees more flexion than the limits of the contracture. The greater contracture and the longer the residual limb, the more problems of socket construction. A balance exists between involuntary and voluntary knee control. The more involuntary knee control, the greater stance stability; however, initiating knee flexion on swinging becomes more difficult. More active individuals require a minimum of involuntary knee control to maintain as much voluntary control of knee action as possible. Knee control varies with hydraulic or stance support knee mechanisms. See Chapter 7 for details of these components.

Transfemoral Gait Analysis

NORMAL PROSTHETIC GAIT

Heel Contact to Midstance, Lateral View

The knee is in extension from heel contact to midstance as the foot descends smoothly to the floor and the weight of the body progresses easily to a balanced point over the support leg. The body moves forward and slightly laterally to achieve this position.

T A B L E   8 . 2   **STATIC TRANSFEMORAL PROSTHETIC EVALUATION**

Checkout Item	What to Check	Possible Problem
Before Donning		
Is the inside of the socket smoothly finished?	Feel the inside of the socket.	Skin abrasions.
Does the socket meet socket specification (e.g., ischial containment or quadrilateral)?	Compare with prescription.	
Do all joints move freely and smoothly?	Check particularly the hip and knee joints.	Joints that are too stiff or too loose cause gait deviations.
Sitting		
Is the socket securely on the residual limb?	Pull on the socket slightly.	Suspension should be maintained in all positions.
Does the length of the shin and thigh correspond to the length of shin and thigh of the unamputated leg?	Check to see that the knees are level when the client is sitting with the knee flexed to 90 degrees.	A high prosthetic knee could indicate a misaligned knee joint and lead to poor swing-through.
Can the client sit comfortably, without burning or pinching?	Check the posterior wall, particularly the pressure of the posterior brim against the seat and residual limb.	A sharp posterior wall can cause sciatic nerve pressure.
Is the client able to lean forward and reach her or his shoes?	Check the anterior wall height when sitting.	The anterior wall may impinge on the abdominal area.
Standing		
Does the socket fit properly and comfortably?	Ask the client if he or she is comfortable.	Areas of discomfort can cause gait deviations, failure to wear the prosthesis, and skin problems.
Is the knee stable when weight is placed on the prosthesis?	The knee joint is initially aligned on or just behind a line dropped from the trochanter to the knee axis. If the knee is in front of the line, it will be unstable.	An unstable knee can lead to an insecure gait.
Is the pelvis level when weight is borne evenly on both legs?	Palpate both iliac crests with the client standing with weight equally distributed on the two legs.	A prosthesis that is too long or too short will lead to gait deviations.
Does the socket maintain good contact with the residual limb on all sides as the client shifts weight?	Check the brim of the socket as the client shifts weight.	A socket that is too loose or too tight may lead to skin abrasions and discomfort.
Is there an adductor roll?	Check high in the groin for excessive tissue around the medial wall.	An adductor roll can be pinched between the top of the medial wall and the pubic ramus leading to pain and an abducted gait.
Is there pressure on the pubic ramus?	Ask the client.	Pain can lead to an abducted gait.

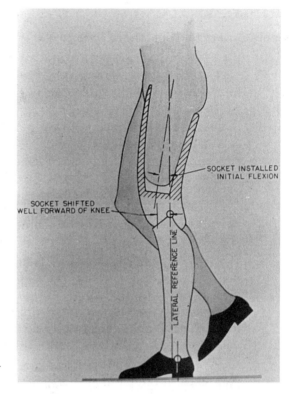

SOCKET INSTALLED
INITIAL FLEXION

SOCKET SHIFTED
WELL FORWARD OF KNEE

LATERAL REFERENCE LINE

FIGURE 8.22
The trochanter knee ankle line (lateral reference line).

Midstance, Anterior View

There may be a slight pelvic drop, less than 5 degrees and no more than 2.5 centimeters lateral trunk bending. The individual exhibits good medial lateral stability and balance on the prosthesis as the contralateral foot is picked up for swing phase. The width of the gait base should not exceed 5 centimeters.

Midstance to Toe Off, Lateral View

Heel rise is smooth as the weight is brought forward over the prosthetic forefoot. The hip extends without lumbar lordosis and the knee begins to flex as the toe leaves the ground.

Swing Phase, Lateral View

The foot leaves the ground. The prosthetic knee bends smoothly. The hip and knee flex as the prosthetic leg swings forward in the line of progression. Heel rise is adequate for the prosthetic toe to clear the floor but is not excessive. The shank swings smoothly and quietly forward and the knee is extended just before the next heel contact. The stride length is equal on both sides.

TRANSFEMORAL GAIT DEVIATIONS

Heel Contact to Midstance, Lateral View

Knee Instability Knee instability is the major problem that can occur between heel contact and midstance (Fig. 8.23). It is essential for the knee to be extended for the client to feel secure. Causes of knee instability include:

1   If the knee axis is placed anterior to the TKA line, the line of body weight falls behind the knee, creating a flexion moment. The knee can be malaligned if the socket is placed too far anterior (long heel lever arm).
2   Knee instability can also be caused by lack of adequate socket flexion limiting the client's active hip extension.
3   A heel cushion that is too hard and does not accept body weight may also create a flexion moment at heel strike.
4   A severe hip flexion contracture not accommodated in the socket makes it difficult for the client to control the knee.

Terminal Impact This term refers to a rapid forward movement of the shank that allows the knee to reach maximum extension with too much force before heel strike. It occurs most frequently in prostheses with constant friction knees in which the client uses sound to indicate that the knee is ready for heel contact. It is a difficult habit to change. The impact, if severe, can cause bruising of the distal end of the residual limb. It does not occur with properly functioning hydraulic knee mechanisms.

Foot Slap If the forefoot descends too rapidly, it will make a slapping sound as it hits the floor (Fig. 8.24). This may be caused by plantar flexion resistance that is too soft or a heel lever arm that is too short. The client may also be driving

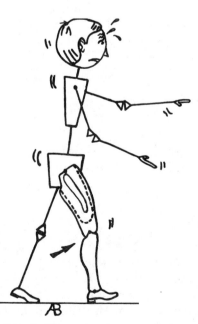

FIGURE 8.23
Heel contact to midstance: knee instability. (Artist: Angie Britt)

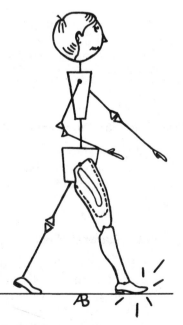

FIGURE 8.24
Heel contact to midstance: foot slap. (Artist: Angie Britt)

the prosthesis into the walking surface too forcibly to ensure extension of the knee. It is not a frequent problem.

Midstance, Anterior/Posterior View

Lateral Trunk Bending   All individuals walking with a transfemoral prosthesis exhibit some lateral bending from the midline to the prosthetic side because the prosthesis cannot fully compensate for loss of skeletal fixation to the ground (Fig. 8.25). Excessive bending may have several causes:

1   The lateral wall of the socket is designed to provide mediolateral stability by holding the limb in adduction. If the residual limb is short, or if adduction of the socket is inadequate, there will be lateral trunk bending at midstance.

2   A prosthesis that is too short will cause a hip drop at midstance, as well as lateral trunk bending.

3   If the medial wall of the socket is too high, the client may bend laterally to avoid discomfort.

4   The client may not have adequate balance to properly shift the weight over the prosthesis or may have a short residual limb that fails to provide a sufficient lever arm for the pelvis.

5   The client may have weak abductors on the prosthetic side and be unable to control the body weight over the prosthesis.

6   This gait deviation may also be seen if the client's residual limb is producing pain.

Abducted Gait   An abducted gait is characterized by a gait base that is wider than 5 centimeters at midstance (Fig. 8.26). Causes include:

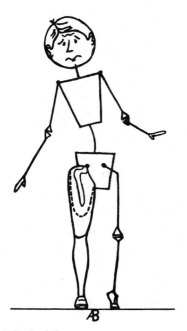

FIGURE 8.25
Midstance: lateral trunk bending to prosthetic side. (Artist: Angie Britt)

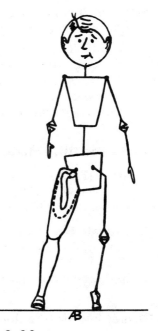

FIGURE 8.26
Midstance: abducted gait. (Artist: Angie Britt)

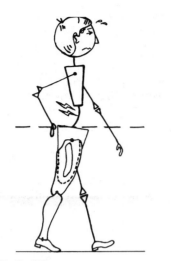

FIGURE 8.27
Midstance to toe off: lumbar lordosis. (Artist: Angie Britt)

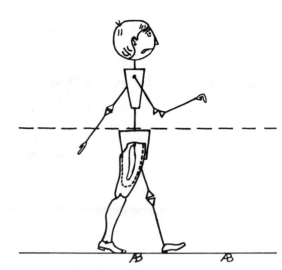

FIGURE 8.28
Terminal stance: drop off. (Artist: Angie Britt)

1   A prosthesis that is too long.
2   An improperly shaped lateral wall that fails to provide adequate support for the femur.
3   A high medial wall that causes the client to hold the prosthesis away to avoid ramus pressure.
4   The pelvic band may be positioned too far away from the patient's body.
5   The client may have an abduction contracture or have developed a poor gait pattern.

Extensive Trunk Extension   Some clients may extend the trunk excessively from heel contact to midstance (Fig. 8.27).

1   Insufficient initial socket flexion leads the client to extend the lumbar spine to obtain hip extension necessary for knee control.
2   The client may have a flexion contracture that cannot be accommodated prosthetically.
3   The client may have weak hip extensors or abdominals.

Midstance to Toe Off, Lateral View

Drop Off (Fig. 8.22)   As with the transtibial prosthesis, there is a sudden downward movement of the trunk as anterior support is lost prematurely (Fig. 8.28). The main reason is usually a toe lever arm that is too short.

Inadequate Heel Off   If the client does not feel secure in allowing the body weight to shift forward over the toe of the prosthesis, the heel may not come off the floor until the whole foot is brought forward. This deviation is associated with uneven steps, discussed later in this chapter.

Swing Phase, Anterior/Posterior View

Circumducted Gait   During circumducted gait, the prosthesis swings laterally in an arclike manner during swing phase. Causes include:

1 A prosthesis that is too long.

2 A mechanical knee with too much alignment stability or friction in the knee, making it difficult to bend the knee in swing through.

3 The client may not be confident about flexing the prosthetic knee because of muscle weakness or fear of stubbing the toe.

4 The stance phase control knee may not be functioning properly.

Vaulting The client rises on the toe of the sound foot to swing the prosthesis through with little knee flexion. Some individuals use this maneuver temporarily to walk rapidly. Unwanted or continuous vaulting may be caused by:

1 A prosthesis that is too long.

2 Inadequate socket suspension.

3 Excessive stability in the alignment or some limitation of knee flexion such as a knee lock.

4 Fear of stubbing the toe or flexing the knee may cause this defect, or it may be related to discomfort.

Medial or Lateral Whips Whips (Fig. 8–29) are best observed when the client walks away from the observer. A medial whip is present when the heel travels medially on initial flexion at the beginning of swing phase; a lateral whip exists when the heel moves laterally. Prosthetically, whips are always related to the knee joint.

1 Medial whips result from excessive external rotation of the prosthetic knee.

2 Lateral whips result from excessive internal rotation of the prosthetic knee.

3 Other causes may include a socket that is too tight, reflecting residual limb rotation, or the client may have donned the prosthesis in internal or external rotation.

Uneven Arm Swing and Uneven Timing These two deviations are seen together. The arm on the prosthetic side is held close to the body and the individual takes steps of unequal duration and length with a short stance phase on

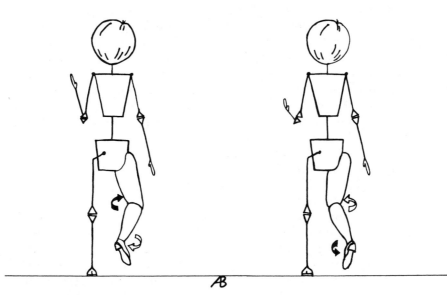

FIGURE 8.29
Swing phase: *(left)* medial heel whip; *(right)* lateral heel whip. (Artist: Angie Britt)

prosthesis. The major causes are poor training and fear of putting weight on the prosthesis.

Basic Gait Training

CASE STUDY ACTIVITIES

1 Design a prosthetic training program for each client. What do you already know? What do you need to learn?
2 Compare and contrast prosthetic training programs for a person fitted with a transtibial prosthesis and another fitted with an transfemoral prosthesis.
3 What parts of training are appropriately done by a PTA?

Donning the Prosthesis

Proper prosthetic donning is one of the first things to be learned. Teaching proper donning method involves showing the client the appropriate reference points between the residual limb and the socket and having the client learn the correct feel of the prosthesis. Sockets that fit snugly (e.g., some suction prostheses) are more difficult to don.

RESIDUAL LIMB SOCK

Most prostheses are worn with a sock that fits directly over the residual limb and is applied before the residual limb is inserted in the socket. In all but suction sockets, the sock remains as an additional interface while the prosthesis is worn. Socks come in different thicknesses or plys. A thin cotton sock is considered to be one ply; wool socks are made in either three or five ply. Some clients with bony or sensitive residual limbs may choose to wear a thin nylon sheath under the cotton or wool sock to reduce skin friction during ambulation. Individuals whose residual limbs have difficulty tolerating the stresses of active prosthetic wear, including some athletes, may wear a gel impregnated sheath that provides additional shock absorption. The mineral oil gel is on the lower half of the sheath. Nylon and gel sheaths are worn directly over the residual limb. The nylon sheath is equal to less than a single ply, but the gel impregnated sheath is equivalent to a two ply sock distally. Initial prosthetic fitting is made with either a one or three ply sock. As the residual limb shrinks, additional socks must be added. Socks and sheaths come in a variety of sizes and widths for both transtibial and transfemoral residual limbs. During initial training, the PT or PTA emphasizes that the sock must be pulled over the residual limb completely with the distal seam running parallel to the incision line in a mediolateral direction. Care must be taken that the sock is smooth and unwrinkled. The PT or PTA teaches the client how to adjust socks as the residual limb shrinks, as discussed later in this chapter. Figure 8.30 illustrates several types of residual limb socks and replacement sheaths. Figure 8.31 is a client education handout on the selection, fit, and care of residual limb socks.

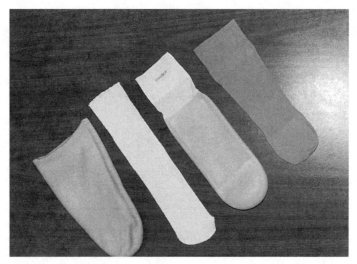

FIGURE 8.30
Residual limb socks and sheaths. From the bottom left: a five ply wool sock, a one ply cotton sock, a Silosheath (Silipos Corporation), and a nylon sheath.

SYME'S AND TRANSTIBIAL PROSTHESES

The residual limb fits snugly into the socket with its distal end touching the distal end pad in transtibial prostheses and with some end bearing in a Syme's leg. At both levels, the patellar bar presses the midline of the patella tendon. Because some prostheses are designed to fit snugly, the client may have to stand to get the residual limb completely into the socket. Care must be taken not to abrade the skin when donning the prosthesis. On occasion, clients may experience some difficulty donning a prosthesis with high medial and lateral walls; a slight turning of the residual limb as the prosthesis is being donned will ease the tibial condyles past the wings of the prosthesis. Suspension straps are secured after the residual limb is well into the socket. If a liner is worn, it can be donned first, then the residual limb and liner are inserted into the socket (Fig. 8.32). This process may be difficult for clients with impaired balance or impaired vision. Fitting the liner and socket separately may increase the likelihood of an improperly donned prosthesis. It may be easier to teach the client to put the socket and liner on as a single unit.

TRANSFEMORAL PROSTHESES

When the client dons the ischial containment socket, care must be taken to ensure that the socket is not rotated internally or externally. The lateral wall and foot position are guides to proper donning (Fig. 8.33). In the quadrilateral socket, the adductor longus channel at the anteromedial corner of the socket and the ischial seat on top of the posterior wall are major reference points. Transfemoral prostheses with pelvic band suspension are usually donned in the sitting position, while the suction sockets are donned standing.

The suction transfemoral prosthesis is worn without a sock; a stockinet or elastic bandage is used to pull the residual limb into the socket and push the

PROPER USE OF SOCKS FOR YOUR RESIDUAL LIMB

Socks are worn over your residual limb within the prosthetic socket unless you have been fitted with a suction type of prosthetic socket. The sock is designed to increase the comfort of the prosthetic socket and to assist in control of perspiration. The socks allow you to maintain a close socket fit as your residual limb shrinks.

Socks come in different lengths, widths, thicknesses, and materials. Your socks have been selected to fit your particular residual limb. No other type of residual limb cover will fit properly, and only these socks should be used over your residual limb when wearing your prosthesis. The thickness of the residual limb sock is called a "ply." Thin or cotton socks are considered one-ply. Your initial fit may be with a single one-ply or thin sock. Thicker socks are made of wool and are generally either three-ply or five-ply. Socks come in other thicknesses for special needs, but most clients receive a number of thin or one-ply socks and three three-ply and three five-ply socks. Three-and five-ply socks in cotton are available for individuals who are allergic to wool but are not recommended for general use.

Putting on the Socks Properly

Pull sock on firmly, without leaving any wrinkles. The seam at the end of the sock should run parallel to, not across, the suture line. Put on clean, dry socks each day, because wet or dirty socks can cause injury to the residual limb. If you are wearing more than one sock over your residual limb, put each one on separately, making sure it fits snugly and has no wrinkles.

Care of the Socks

Wash wool socks by hand with mild soap; rinse well and dry flat. Do not place in the washing machine or dryer. Cotton socks and socks made from acrylic may be machine washed in cold water and dried at low temperatures.

Adjusting Socks

A snug, comfortable fit between the residual limb and the socket is necessary to prevent injury to your residual limb. A good fit includes contact between your residual limb and the bottom of the socket. As your residual limb gets smaller (shrinks), you may feel you are going too deep in the socket and may feel excess pressure at the distal end or on a bony prominence at the top of the socket. The socket may also feel loose. If your socket feels loose or if you feel excess pressure at the bottom of the socket, add one thin sock. It may be necessary to add a second thin sock if the first does not relieve the symptoms. Be careful of adding too many socks and thereby pushing your residual limb out of the socket. Add only one sock at a time and check the fit of the socket each time. You may substitute a three-ply sock (with the yellow band at the top) for three cotton socks, or a five-ply (with the green band at the top) for five cotton socks. Some people need to add a sock in the middle of the day after wearing the prosthesis for several hours.

Sheaths

You may wish to don a thin nylon sheath directly over the residual limb before donning the regular socks. Some people prefer the sheath because it can reduce possible friction between the socket and the residual limb and thus provide a smoother interface. A gel-impregnated sheath is also available to provide additional cushioning.

Removing Socks

Some people gain weight after they have been fitted with a prosthesis; others have fluctuations in the size of their residual limb. Wearing too many socks pushes your residual limb out of the socket so that you will no longer be in contact with the bottom. After you have worn a prosthesis for several months, your residual limb will stabilize and you will not need to add or remove socks unless your weight changes or you have major fluctuations in bodily fluids. If you have any questions about proper use of socks, ask your prosthetist or physical therapist.

FIGURE 8.31
Client education handout on the proper use of socks for the residual limb.

air out of the socket at the same time. The skin of the residual limb must be dry and free from abrasions. The wrap is put on the residual limb smoothly and without wrinkles as far as the groin; maintaining all weight on the sound leg, the end is placed through the hole at the end of the socket. The client then stands, places the prosthesis slightly in front of the other leg, then flexes and extends the sound hip and knee while pulling downward on the end of the

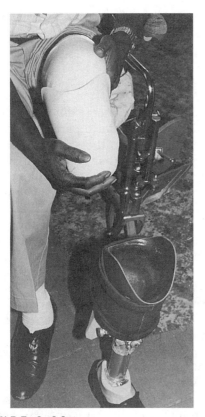

FIGURE 8.32
Donning the patellar socket bearing liner before donning the prosthesis. The residual limb is covered by a sock.

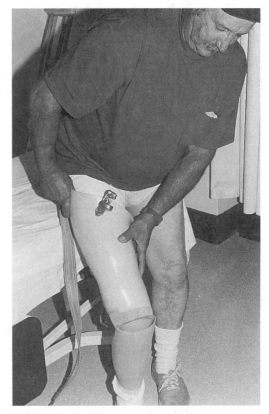

FIGURE 8.33
Donning a transfemoral prosthesis with an ischial containment socket suspended by a Silesian bandage.

wrap. In this manner the residual limb is pulled into the socket and the air is pushed out. The process is continued until the residual limb is in the socket and the wrap has been removed. The valve is then replaced and any remaining air is expelled by shifting all body weight into the prosthesis while holding the valve stem open. If a Silesian bandage is worn, it is secured at this time (see Fig. 7.21). The client learns to carry a pull wrap at all times in case the prosthesis is removed for any reason. Donning a suction socket takes balance and coordination; not all clients like the process. In warm, humid climates, perspiration makes donning and maintaining suction difficult.

HIP DISARTICULATION AND HEMIPELVECTOMY PROSTHESES

These prostheses can be donned either sitting or standing. Most of the body weight is borne on the sound side and the socket is slipped into place. After standing, the client tightens the straps and adjusts them for comfort. The major reference points are the iliac crest and ischium on the amputated side for hip disarticulation or the contralateral iliac crest and ribs for hemipelvectomy prostheses. Instead of socks, many clients prefer to sew the bottom of a T shirt together on the amputated side and slide it over the residual limb. This maneuver limits bunching of fabric that can cause pressure points.

Prosthetic Training

The major goal of prosthetic rehabilitation is a smooth, energy efficient gait that allows the client to perform activities of daily living and to participate in desired work and recreation. The term **mobility** refers to the skills required to solve movement problems confronted during activities. The client is an integral part of the prosthetic training program and helps establish goals. Clients who have functioned with a diseased limb for a considerable period of time frequently exceed their premorbid level of function.

Factors that contribute to a smooth, energy efficient gait include the ability to: (1) accept the weight of the body on each leg; (2) balance on one foot in single limb support; (3) advance each limb forward and prepare for the next step; and (4) adapt to environmental demands. Traditional prosthetic training has focused on breaking down the gait cycle into smaller steps and then teaching each step. Normal gait is an integrated activity that may not be learned most efficiently through the practice of each part. Dennis and McKeough[13] developed a taxonomy of motor tasks based on the work of Gentile[14] that describes environmental conditions involved in regaining independent function. The taxonomy is easily applicable to the clinical setting and provides a reference point for organizing and sequencing patient activities.

Figure 8.34 is a schematic representation of the Dennis and McKeough taxonomy as a two dimensional grid. One dimension (the horizontal axis of the grid) represents desired outcomes, progressing from simple goals requiring body stability (e.g., sitting or standing) to more demanding goals requiring transporting the body through space and time (e.g., walking). Both classes of outcomes—body stability and body in motion—are subdivided into two further classifications: goals that do not require manipulation (e.g., reaching for an object) and those that do. The result is four categories of goals ranged along the horizontal axis and progressing from simple on the left to more demanding on the right. Similarly, the vertical axis of the grid represents variables in environment, with the less demanding environmental situations at the top and the more demanding at the bottom. The two primary categories in the environmental dimension are closed and open. A closed environment, for example, a room with furniture but no people, is one that does not change during performance of the desired goal. An open environment, for instance, a room with a baby on the floor or an elevator, is one that changes during task performance. Again, each major category is subdivided into two variables: in one, there is no variation in the environment between trials (i.e., the space remains the same each time the client attempts a goal); in the other, more difficult variable, the environment changes between trials (e.g., the width of doorways or the placement of furniture may change). As with the horizontal axis, the categories on the vertical axis are arranged in order of increasing difficulty, in this case, from the simplest at the top to the most demanding at the bottom.

These concepts can guide the therapist in planning the sequence of training activities. The training program starts in a closed environment with stability, then mobility activities and progresses to the more complex open environment.

	BODY STABLE		BODY TRANSPORT	
	Without Manipulation	With Manipulation	Without Manipulation	With Manipulation
CLOSED ENVIRONMENT Without Intertrial Variability	Body is stable, arms and legs are still, the task does not change, the environment is fixed in time & space.	Body is stable, task does not change, environment is fixed in time & space, arms or legs are moving,	Body is moving, limbs moving in relation to movement task, task does not change, environment is fixed in time & space	Body is moving, arms or legs moving independently of task, environment is fixed in time & space
With Intertrial Variability	As above but task changes require slight modification in motor plan from trial to trial	As above but task changes require slight modification of motor plan from trial to trial.	As above but task changes require slight modification of motor plan from trial to trial.	As above but task changes require slight modification of motor plan from trial to trial.
OPEN ENVIRONMENT Without Intertrial Variability	Body is stable, arms & legs are still, task is fixed, environment is changing in time & space	Body is stable, task is fixed, arms & legs are moving independently of tasks, environment is changing in time & space	Body is moving, task is fixed, arms and legs and synchronous with task, environment is changing in time & space.	Body is moving, arms or legs moving independently of task, task is fixed, environment changing in time & space.
With Intertrial Variability	As above, but task changes each trial.	As above, but task changes each trial	As above, but task changes each trial	As above but task changes each trial

FIGURE 8.34

Taxonomy of motor tasks: dimensions of task difficulty. (Adapted from Dennis, JK, and McKeough, DM: Mobility. In May, BJ: Home Health and Rehabilitation: Concepts of Care. FA Davis, Philadelphia, 1993.)

As success is achieved at one level, activities can be made more complex by varying the independent limb or by adding intertrial variability.

TEACHING PROSTHETIC CONTROL

Before an individual can develop a smooth, energy efficient gait, he or she must be able to balance on the prosthesis long enough to bring the other leg forward in a controlled manner. Early training starts in a closed environment with little independent limb manipulation. Activities that require side to side weight shifting, one legged standing, reaching for objects in different directions, and forward and back stepping with one foot help the client learn basic prosthetic control and the ''feel'' of the prosthesis when the weight is shifted to different parts of the foot (Fig. 8.35). Reaching for an object in different locations helps the client shift weight on and off the prosthesis in a functional manner (Fig. 8.36). Individuals with transtibial prostheses must learn to let the knee flex

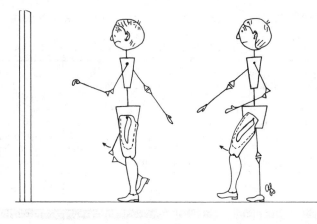

A

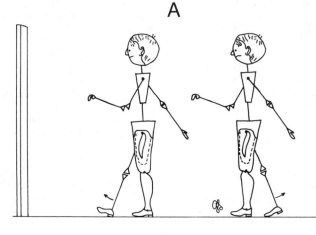

B

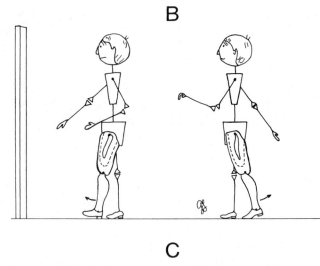

C

FIGURE 8.35
Early prosthetic training. (*A*) Weight shifting on and off the prosthesis, to increase knee control. (*B*) Stepping forward and back with the sound leg increases weight bearing on the prosthesis. (*C*) Alternating stepping forward and back with the prosthesis can increase knee control in swing phase. (Kicking a soft ball enhances both activities shown in *B* and *C*.) (Artist: Gloria Sanders)

slightly from heel strike to midstance in a natural gait pattern. Individuals fitted with transfemoral prostheses need to learn to control the prosthetic knee as part of the initial balancing activities. The PT or PTA can provide some kinesthetic feedback by pushing slightly on the back of the prosthetic knee when the client

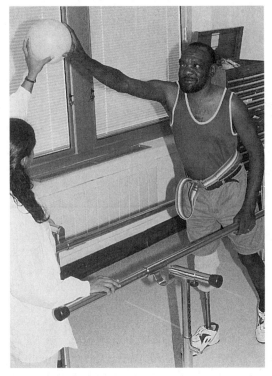

FIGURE 8.36
Reaching for an object promotes weight shifting on and off the prosthesis.

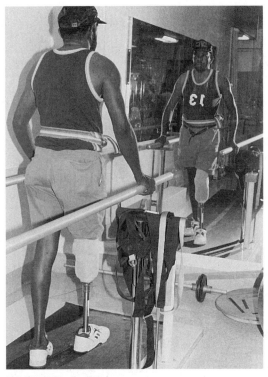

FIGURE 8.37
Training in front of a mirror reduces the tendency to look at the floor.

is in the parallel bars. The client extends the residual limb against the posterior wall of the socket and begins to feel how to control the knee.

Clients often tend to look at the floor during initial training because they cannot feel the floor directly. A mirror helps the person keep the head erect and focus on feeling the socket pressures change during the different parts of weight shifting (Fig. 8.37). Focusing on achieving the goals of an activity such as touching a ball or reaching into a cabinet helps prevent looking at the feet. The ability to shift weight and balance on the prosthesis is critical to a satisfactory gait for all prosthetic wearers. Throughout, the client, as an integral part of the team, needs to learn to give personal feedback on the performance. Asking the client, "How did that feel?" "What would help you make the performance feel natural?" is helpful.

INITIAL WALKING

Energy efficiency is a very important consideration in prosthetic training. The more energy it takes to walk, the less likely the client will do it. Time spent guiding the client to learn good balance, weight shifting, and the initial gait pattern is time well spent. Walking is initiated in the safety of the parallel bars or in a secure area in the home. A mirror may help the person assume a better standing position with the weight well distributed over the feet. Figure 8.38 depicts an initial walking sequence with a transfemoral prosthesis. The individual with a transtibial prosthesis follows a similar sequence but must be re-

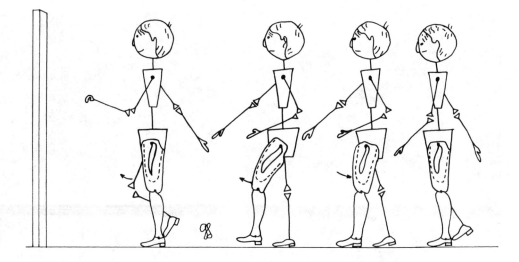

FIGURE 8.38
Learning to walk forward in a coordinated manner using minimal external support if possible. (Artist: Gloria Sanders)

minded to roll over the foot, allowing the knee to flex after midstance. Throughout the early training sequence, the client should be encouraged to put as little weight on the parallel bars as possible, particularly if independent ambulation without external support or with only a cane is anticipated. During initial walking, the PT or PTA can provide feedback based on observation of the gait pattern, suggesting possible changes in movements that may improve the pattern. However, some people cannot benefit from suggestions regarding individual movements. They may develop an awkward gait pattern trying to emphsize what has been suggested, such as taking a longer step with the unamputated leg and shifting weight over the prosthesis more. In some instances, particularly with older people, suggesting that they try to walk "like you did before you lost your leg" is helpful. When the pattern is particularly smooth, asking them "How did that feel?" helps them reintegrate normal movements into their activities. PTs and PTAs are sometimes reluctant to spend adequate time in balance and initial walking. The limited time allowed for rehabilitation by third-party payers sometimes drives the PT to accept a less than desirable gait pattern or reliance on a greater level of external support.

One of the more difficult parts of walking is learning to shift the weight to the prosthesis in a smooth pattern on each step. The creative therapist finds many ways to lead the client to make these movements. Tapping on the side of the hip may help with sideways weight shifting. Occasionally, having the client hold the bar or a cane on the amputated side for several steps may encourage weight shifting (Fig. 8.39). In the home, incorporating everyday activities such as reaching for something on a high shelf, making a bed, or wiping a counter encourages prosthetic weight shifting in a functional pattern (Fig. 8.40). It is important for the client to make a direct transition from the parallel bars to the anticipated final external support. Effective gait training encourages the least amount of external support necessary.

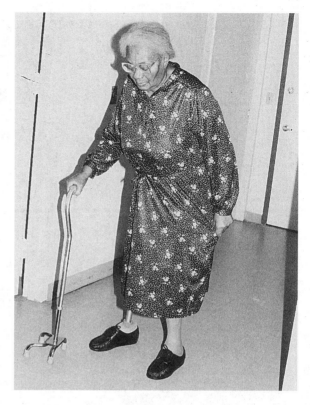

FIGURE 8.39
Sometimes using the cane on the prosthetic side helps the client learn to weight shift to that side.

Integration of the prosthesis into a variety of gait situations is important; learning to sidestep and walk backwards is helpful to provide weight shifting, prosthetic control, balance, and function (Fig. 8.41). During the initial training, the person must be taught a safe way to get up and down from a chair (Fig. 8.42). Figure 8.43 illustrates the use of the Dennis and McKeough taxonomy to progress training activities.

HYDRAULIC KNEE MECHANISMS

Many different knee mechanisms are in use throughout the United States. The PT and PTA become familiar with the devices in use in their regions through regular contact with local prosthetists. Training an individual fitted with a hydraulic knee mechanism is somewhat different from training one fitted with a mechanical knee joint. In all models, the hydraulic mechanism is designed for swing phase control and adjusts the swing of the shank to ensure that the foot is ready for heel strike at the appropriate time. Rather than increasing or decreasing hip flexion force to adjust shank swing, the person lets the hydraulic mechanism do the job. The client needs to experience different cadences to understand the capabilities of hydraulic swing phase control.

The Mauch S-N-S (M+IND Corp) and other swing and stance phase control systems require different training for knee control. The system has three modes: swing and stance phase control, swing phase control only, and knee flexion lock. For the system to be operational, the client must be taught to walk over

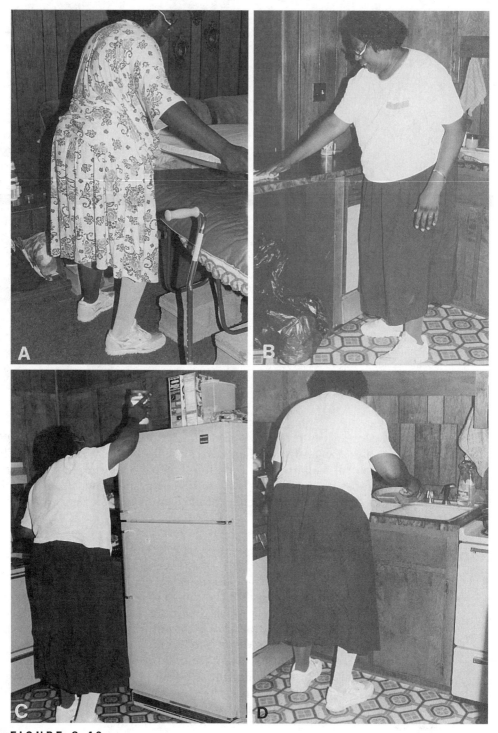

FIGURE 8.40
Prosthetic training in the home: incorporating functional activities increases the internalization of prosthetic use.

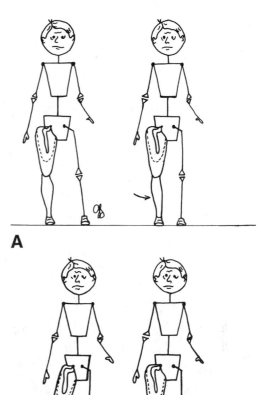

FIGURE 8.41
Prosthetic training: learning to step sideways.
(Artist: Gloria Sanders)

A

B

the ball of the foot. Putting pressure on the ball of the foot allows the knee to flex naturally. Active individuals gain control easily, but more timid walkers may have difficulty initiating knee flexion.

EXTERNAL SUPPORT

Energy expenditure is a major concern; it is directly related to the smoothness of the gait pattern and the use of external devices. It is desirable to train the person to functional ambulation without using external devices. A single point or quad cane is often needed by elderly people for use in the street. On occasion, crutches may be needed if the client has other medical conditions that preclude ambulating with less support. A four point gait is usually taught unless the client needs to protect the unamputated leg from full weight bearing (Fig. 8.44). A walker is not indicated in most instances and should not be considered as an intermediate phase between the parallel bars and a cane. A walker does not allow a smooth step over step pattern and reinforces a slow gait pattern char-

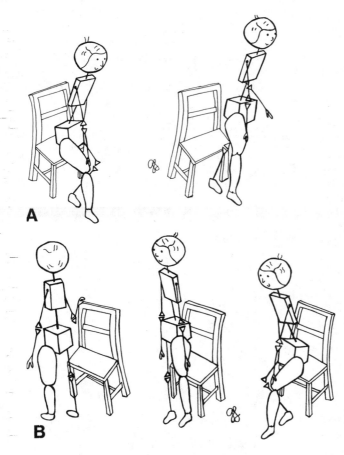

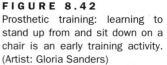

FIGURE 8.42
Prosthetic training: learning to stand up from and sit down on a chair is an early training activity. (Artist: Gloria Sanders)

acterized by uneven steps. This gait negates the principles of prosthetic design and alignment. The walker also reinforces forward flexion and eliminates the normal use of the arms in the gait pattern. Using the walker as a shortcut to allow the client to be discharged from treatment early or to use the prosthesis at home before a good gait has been achieved leads to gait deviations and a dependence on the walker that may never be overcome. A walker should be used *only* if it is obvious that the individual will not be able to use the prosthesis with any other form of external support. An elderly person who can go to the bathroom independently with a walker is easier to care for at home than one who depends on a wheelchair. The walker should, however, be used sparingly and only after careful evaluation of the individual's potential.

ADVANCED TRAINING

CASE STUDY ACTIVITIES

1 Design training programs for Diana Magnolia and Ha Lee Davis that incorporate progression from a closed to an open environment.
2 Identify at least two activities for each cell of the models that you would perform in a rehabilitation center and in a home.

Changing the environment is an integral part of the gait training program. It is hardly functional to have the client walk only in the sheltered and simple

		BODY STABLE		BODY TRANSPORT	
		Without Manipulation	With Manipulation	Without Manipulation	With Manipulation
CLOSED	Without Intertrial Variability	Keeps balance standing while PT/PTA gently and predictably pushes on body	Dons prosthesis in sitting or standing position. Stands and reaches for object with 1 or 2 hands	Rolling over in bed; sit to stand from bed or wheelchair using cane, crutches, or wheelchair.	Carries the same object from place to place using same pathway. Sit to stand with an object in hand (not a walking aid).
	With Intertrial Variability	Keeps sitting or standing balance on different surfaces e.g. carpet, tiles, straight chair, sofa, etc.	Stands at a counter reaching for different objects placed in different positions. Sits, bends and reaches for object	Sit to stand from different surfaces and different height chairs. Up and down curbs of different heights	Carries objects of different size and weight from place to place using different pathways.
OPEN	Without Intertrial Variability	Keeps balance in a moving elevator or a moving platform	Rearranges packages in a moving elevator. Handles several objects while standing on an unstable surface.	Walks down a hallway with the same person coming toward them.	Carries an object while walking down the hallway.
	With Intertrial Variability	Keeps balance while catching and throwing a ball	Stands in a crowded room, eating or drinking from glass or plate in hand.	Community ambulation; walks through a busy gym.	Shops in a supermarket; goes to a room, picks up some objects, walks back through busy hallway.

FIGURE 8.43
Using the taxonomy of motor skills to prioritize training activities. (Adapted from Dennis, JK, and Mc-Keough, DM: Mobility. In May, BJ: Home Health and Rehabilitation: Concepts of Care. FA Davis, Philadelphia, 1993.)

environment of the physical therapy gym. Functional ambulation takes place in both complex closed environments and open environments. It is the responsibility of the PT and PTA to provide opportunities to practice these skills. Walking around furniture, through narrow doorways, on rugs, and around obstacles is very different from walking in the gym. Although this is still a closed environment because there are no moving objects requiring predictive ability, it is more complex than on wide pathways without obstacles. Placing obstacles on the floor to step around or over or walking in a busy hallway of the treatment centers are progression activities. The home environment is also replete with opportunities for such progression. An even more complex closed environment

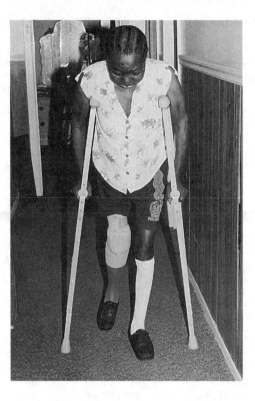

FIGURE 8.44
Some clients need to limit weight bearing on the sound leg; this can be done using the four point gait with crutches.

is created by having the client pick something up from the floor or carry an object in one hand (Fig. 8.45 and 8.46). These activities require balance, coordination, and the ability to shift weight on and off the prosthesis in different body positions. It becomes an open environment activity when other people are in the room or hall (Fig. 8.47).

During advanced training the client is taught a safe way to get up and down from chairs of different heights and different degrees of seat resilience, especially toilet seats.

Care of the Prosthesis, Residual Limb, and Socks

Teaching the client proper care of the residual limb and how to adjust socks is an integral part of the training program. The PT and PTA should contact the prosthetist to learn proper care of the particular materials used in the prosthesis. Most plastic sockets and liners can be washed with a damp cloth and dried thoroughly. The socket should be washed at night to allow plenty of time for it to dry. Socks must also be washed and changed daily. Wool socks require hand washing with mild soap before they are dried flat. Learning to adjust socks to accommodate a shrinking residual limb or for an individual whose weight fluctuates is more complicated, but it is important that each person understand both the purpose and adjustment of socks. Figure 8.33 contains an example of instructions that can be given to clients on the care of the socks.

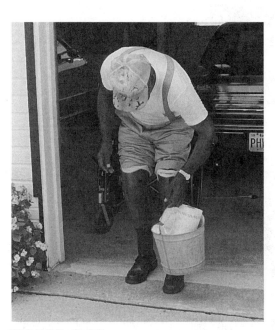

FIGURE 8.45
Learning to pick up an object from the floor requires balance and coordination.

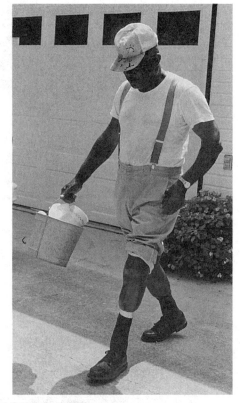

FIGURE 8.46
Carrying an item is an advanced activity requiring independent limb manipulation.

Individuals with Bilateral Prostheses

The basic gait training activities for a person with bilateral prostheses are similar to those used with clients with a single prosthesis. If the individual ambulated with one prosthesis before losing the other limb, the process is easier. Most individuals with two prostheses need some form of external support, especially for elevation activities.

Considerable time needs to be spent on balance and weight shifting activities since the individual no longer has any direct contact with the ground. Individuals with two prostheses use a somewhat wider base of support than those with one prosthesis; many exhibit a tendency to roll a bit from side to side. Although these extraneous movements need to be minimized, they may not be completely eliminated. The client should progress directly from the parallel bars to whatever form of external support will be used at home. A walker is again not the external support of choice. Functional outcomes are directly related to the balance, strength, and coordination of the client and to the level of amputation. The amount of energy expended must not be so great as to preclude participation in other activities. The higher the levels of amputation and the more external support needed, the less functional the ambulation.[7]

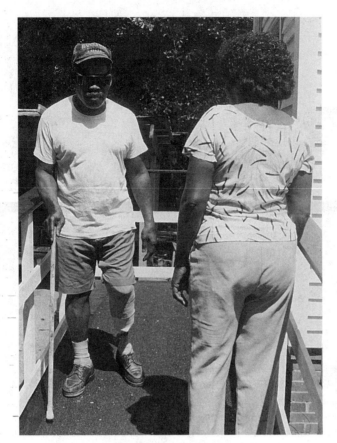

FIGURE 8.47
An open environment type of activity can be created by having a family member walk in front of the client while the client is ambulating in a familiar space.

All individuals with one prosthesis need support for times when they are not wearing the prosthesis; those with two prostheses need a wheelchair with offset wheels or anterior weights to counter the loss of weight in the front of the chair.

SUMMARY

Training the individual to regain independence in mobility with a prosthesis is a sequential program of balance and basic and advanced gait activities. The discharge environment and the client's functional needs and expectations must be considered to plan an effective treatment program. The training program demands creativity from PTs and PTAs, as well as an understanding of motor skills acquisition.

GLOSSARY

Adjuvant therapy	Use of other forms of treatment in addition to the major treatment, usually surgery.
Alignment	Relationship between the different components or parts of the prosthesis in both linear and angular positions.

Doffing	Removing the prosthesis.
Donning	Putting on the prosthesis.
Furuncle	A boil.
Gait cycle	Period between heel contact of one foot and the next heel contact of the same foot. Includes a period of single stance of each foot, a period of double stance, and a period of swing on each leg.
Heel lever arm	Distance from the end of the prosthetic heel to the midpoint of the shoe.
TKA line	A line drawn from the greater trochanter, through the knee axis, to the middle of the ankle. It is used to align the socket to the foot of the prosthesis.
Toe lever arm	Distance from the middle of the prosthetic foot to the end of the toe.
Total contact	The residual limb is in contact with all parts of the socket with appropriate pressure.

REFERENCES

1. Siriwardena, GJA, and Bertrand, PV: Factors influencing rehabilitation of arteriosclerotic lower limb amputees. J Rehab Res 28:35–44, 1991.
2. Steen-Jensen, J, Mandrup-Poulsen, T, and Krasnik, M: Prosthetic fitting in lower limb amputees. Acta Orthop Scand 54:101–103, 1983.
3. Traugh, GH, Corcoran, PJ, and Recess, RL: Energy expenditure of ambulation in patients with transfemoral amputations. Arch Phys Med Rehabil 56:67–71, 1975.
4. Waters, RL, Perry, J, Antonelli, D, and Hislop, H: The energy cost of walking of amputees: Influence of level of amputation. J Bone Joint Surg Am 58:42–46,1976.
5. Jaegers, SMHJ, Vos, LD, Rispens, P, and Hof, AL: The relationship between comfortable and most metabolically efficient walking speed in persons with unilateral above-knee amputation. Arch Phys Med Rehabil 74:521–525, 1993.
6. Waters, RL: The energy expenditure of amputee gait. In Bowker, JH, and Michael, JW (eds.): Atlas of Limb Prosthetics: Surgical, Prosthetic, and Rehabilitation Principles, ed. 2. Mosby-Year Book, St. Louis, 1992, pp. 381–388.
7. Pinzur, MS, Gottschalk, F, Smith, D, et al: Functional outcome of below-knee amputation in peripheral vascular insufficiency: A multicenter review. Clinical Orthop 286:247–249, 1993.
8. Muecke, L, Shekar, S, Dwyer, D, et al: Functional screening of lower-limb amputees: A role in predicting rehabilitation outcome? Arch Phys Med Rehabil 73:851–858, 1992.
9. Nitz, JC: Rehabilitation outcomes after bilateral lower limb amputation for vascular disease. Physiotherapy Theory and Practice 9:165–170, 1993.
10. Nissen, SJ, Newman, WP: Factors influencing reintegration to normal living after amputation. Arch Phys Med Rehabil 73:548–551, 1992.
11. Barbera, J, and Albert-Pampl, R: Centrocentral anastomosis of the proximal nerve stump in the treatment of painful amputation neuromas of major nerves. J Neurosurg 79:331–334, 1993.
12. Perry, J: Normal gait. In Bowker, JH, and Michael, JW (eds.): Atlas of Limb Prosthetics: Surgical, Prosthetic, and Rehabilitation Principles, ed. 2. Mosby-Year Book, St. Louis, 1992, pp. 359–370.
13. Dennis, JK, and McKeough, DM: Mobility. In May, BJ: Home Health and Rehabilitation: Concepts of Care. F A Davis, Philadelphia, 1993, pp. 143–172.
14. Gentile, AM: A working model of skill acquisition with application of teaching. Quest 27:3, 1972.

chapter nine

Long Term Care

OBJECTIVES

At the end of this chapter, all students are expected to:

1   Discuss long term adjustment to living with a prosthesis.

2   Describe methods of teaching activities of daily living (ADL) and instrumental activities of daily living (IADL).

3   Discuss recreational opportunities for clients of all ages.

4   Develop a program to teach the client how to care for the prosthesis and residual limb on a long term basis.

case studies

Diana Magnolia: Now independent in ambulation with her prosthesis and one cane in the physical therapy department, she can go up and down steps with a handrail and can go up and down a curb as high as 8 inches. She has the prosthesis at home and is receiving therapy from a home health care agency.

Ha Lee Davis: Independent with his prosthesis and no external support, he was discharged from active therapy after 2 weeks and is going through a work evaluation program sponsored by the State Vocational Rehabilitation Agency. He comes into the physical therapy department one day to ask if he could learn to run a race with his prosthesis. He says he is interested in getting involved in sports activities but does not know where to turn.

Benny Pearl: Inconsistent in attendance at the outpatient clinic, he spent 2 weeks in the local rehabilitation hospital. He was discharged, able to don and doff the prosthesis independently and walk limitedly around the house with a quad cane. He takes a long step with his prosthesis and a short step with his other foot. His wife reports that he needs help to go up and down the three steps outside his house even with a handrail; he cannot go down the single step into the screened porch that does not have a rail. She states that he also has difficulty getting up and down from the low toilet seat.

Betty Childs: Now returned to school with her prosthesis, which she wears every day for all activities, she is not in any active therapy program but will return to the amputee clinic for follow up.

CASE STUDY ACTIVITIES

1   Discuss each client's possible long term psychosocial and financial adjustments to the loss of a limb.
2   What problems might each person have to face to achieve full return to a meaningful lifestyle?

Learning how to walk with a prosthesis is only one component of rehabilitation. Living with a prosthesis requires making changes in lifestyle and daily habits. The individual must cope with new problems that range from going to the bathroom in the middle of the night to finding gainful employment. Return to a full active life is the goal; the dimensions of that life are defined differently by each individual. For some it includes vigorous vocational and recreational activities; for others it may mean being able to work in the garden or walk across the street to visit neighbors. Regardless of lifestyle, each person with an amputation must cope with many physical, psychological, social, and financial adjustments.[1,2]

Prosthetic Care

A prosthesis, like any other mechanical equipment, requires maintenance. Clients also need to be monitored to ensure they are adding socks as the residual limb reduces in size (see Chap. 8). Prosthetists and amputee clinics establish long term recheck appointments with their clients to ensure proper maintenance of the appliance. Generally, the first reevaluation following discharge from initial training takes place within 1 or 2 months of discharge from therapy. The residual limb is likely to have shrunk, and it is important to ensure the client is adjusting socks appropriately. After the client has integrated prosthetic function into daily life and has stabilized medically and functionally, annual reevaluations can be scheduled.

Ideally, the clinic schedule needs to allow time for a full evaluation by the physical therapist before review by the complete team. The evaluation allows time to explore any problems and to obtain data comparable to those gathered in previous visits. Table 9.1 outlines the major components of a long-term evaluation, which varies with each client, with type of prosthesis, and with cause of amputation. The first prosthesis usually lasts 1 to 2 years, depending on the amount of soft tissue in the residual limb at the time of initial fitting, the activity level of the client, and whether the client gains or loses weight. Weight gain is a major problem. Older individuals or people who do not return to premorbid activity level tend to gain weight. Obviously, the prosthesis does not expand with the residual limb, and the client may soon find that the residual limb no longer fits into the socket. Continued wear in such instances causes skin breakdowns and abrasions.

The prosthesis itself needs to be checked to make sure all components are

T A B L E 9 . 1 **LONG-TERM REEVALUATION**

Interview	Prosthetic wear pattern
	Number of days
	Length of time each day
	Reason for wear pattern
	Comfort level with prosthesis
	Activities performed with or without prosthesis
	Adequacy of sock supply
	General medical health
	Condition of other foot
Residual limb	Skin condition
	Circumference measurements
	Range of motion of proximal joint
	Muscle strength
Nonamputated leg (if dysvascular)	Condition of skin, particularly foot and ankle
	Presence of any sores or ulcers
	Presence of edema
	Gross range of motion of major joints, particularly foot and ankle
	Gross strength of major muscles
Prosthesis	Socket fit and number of plys worn
	Condition of:
	Socket and liner if used
	Suspension
	Joints
	Foot
	Shank or cosmetic cover
Gait pattern	Gait deviations
	Ancillary support used
	Changes since discharge from physical therapy (PT)
Other	Condition of shoe, particularly heel height
	Weight as compared to discharge from PT
	Specific tests required for particular disability

in good condition and functioning properly. Clients need to be encouraged to return to the prosthetist for repairs rather than employing a "do it yourself" approach (Fig. 9.1). Some individuals try to make small repairs themselves (e.g., tacking cuffs to sockets or using regular socks rather than stump socks). Inculcating a positive attitude toward regular prosthetic maintenance leads to a better fit and a more functional prosthesis over a longer period. In time, the client will need a new prosthesis because of residual limb shrinkage, component wear, or both. Although many clients like to continue with the same type of prosthesis, new components that may improve function or comfort should be considered. An individual with a stable residual limb may be ready for suction fitting. Individuals with transfemoral amputations may take advantage of new knee mechanisms. One study recommends allowing the individual to try a new component for a week before making a final decision. Final alignment should not be made for 3 weeks until it is certain the gait has stabilized.[3]

Vocational Adjustment

Many individuals with amputations are able to return to their preamputation employment situation; sometimes a change in assigned work within the same

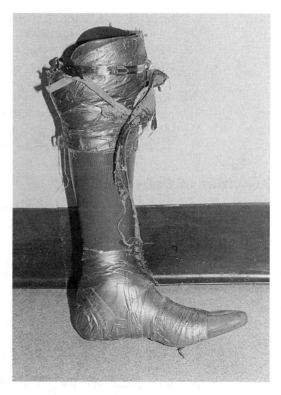

FIGURE 9.1
A "self repaired" prosthesis as it was worn into the clinic.

company is required. A change that leads to lower job status or a decrease in salary tends to increase the person's feelings of inadequacy. For some, a return to preamputation employment is not possible; such individuals must seek other vocational placement. Often it is the less educated and poorer client who has the most difficulty finding gainful employment after amputation. In all states, the Department of Vocational Rehabilitation (different states may have different names) uses federal and state funds to help disabled individuals of working age return to the work force. The help may include providing a prosthesis, rehabilitation, job retraining, and placement. The extent of help available is determined by many factors, including available funds. Despite the Americans with Disabilities Act, which prohibits discrimination on the basis of disability, some employers are reluctant to hire handicapped individuals; counselors from the Department of Vocational Rehabilitation may be helpful. Many factors affect the employability of individuals with amputations, including the national economic status and the attitudes of employers in the community.

Many individuals who undergo lower extremity amputation are retired, either because of a complex of medical problems or because they have reached retirement age. There are as many demands to be met in a satisfactory adaptation to retirement as there are to employment.

CASE STUDY ACTIVITIES

1   Assume you are part of a physical therapist–physical therapist assistant (PT, PTA) team working with Diana Magnolia at home.

Discuss and practice the activities you would teach her to help her reach full independence in all ADL and IADL.

2   How would you answer Ha Lee Davis's questions about running and sports activities? Explore programs and adapted equipment.

3   Assume that you are part of a PT–PTA team working with Benny Pearl in the physical therapy department of a hospital outpatient center. Discuss and practice the activities you would teach him to achieve the goals of getting in and out of his house and using the bathroom safely. Explore the need for special equipment.

Activities of Daily Living

The individual must master many activities after basic walking and climbing stairs have been mastered. Basic ADL include self care and mobility in the home such as walking, using the toilet, getting in and out of a bathtub, and the like. IADL include activities necessary for broad functions such as going shopping, using the phone, and cooking. Advanced activities usually occur in an open environment. Walking on sand, city streets, farm lands, and grass is very different from walking inside a house or therapy department. Learning to cross the street within the green light or "walk" light can be an adventure. The ability to move from place to place independently is of paramount importance in today's lifestyle. Unanticipated barriers can sometimes lead to difficulty; the wise PT or PTA anticipates such barriers and helps the individual learn to surmount them. For example, escalators can seem like mountains when first encountered. A person with relatively good balance can step on and off the escalator with the sound foot on both ascent and descent. Individuals who use crutches or whose balance is not secure are better advised to use elevators. Theater rows or church pews may also represent barriers. The individual needs to be able to sidestep as well as step backwards securely before taking the prosthesis outside. Sidestepping facing the already seated patrons allows the individual to use back and arm rests for any unexpected loss of balance.

ADVANCED ACTIVITIES

Individuals with an amputation below the knee generally learn advanced activities relatively easily. Regardless of the level of amputation, the PT or PTA needs to ensure that the client is able to perform each of these activities—with the possible exception of falling (Figs. 9.2 through 9.5). Depending on the clients' physiological state, balance, and frailty, falling may or may not be practiced. The client needs to be advised to try to fall away from the prosthesis and to put the weight of the body on the uninvolved side. If this activity *is* practiced, it is a good idea to practice falling both forward and backward. Although it is not appropriate to practice falling with all clients, methods of self protection should be discussed routinely. Many elderly individuals who function well without external support in the home need a cane outside the home for extra balance.

Some individuals with one transtibial prosthesis can go up and down stairs one step over the other, depending on the length of the residual limb, the height of the step, and the person's balance and coordination. Extending the knee, as is required by this activity, drives the anterior distal end of the residual limb

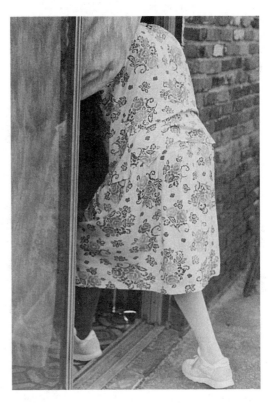

FIGURE 9.2
Independence requires the ability to get into and out of the home.

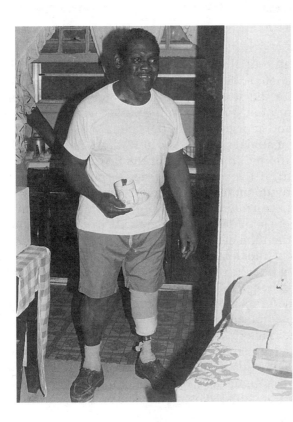

FIGURE 9.3
Carrying an object from room to room enhances balance and coordination training.

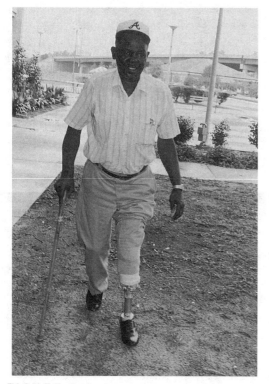

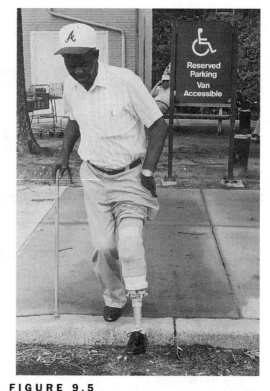

FIGURE 9.4
Learning to walk on uneven ground is part of prosthetic training.

FIGURE 9.5
Crossing the street is a necessary advanced activity.

into the anterior socket wall. Individuals with sensitive skin and poor balance should not attempt this maneuver. Some clients prefer to go up and down steps one at a time, leading with the sound leg going up and with the prosthesis coming down. The amount of advanced training varies with the level of amputation and the balance and coordination of the client.

Most people with a transtibial prosthesis can walk on ramps and inclines with little difficulty. The limited dorsiflexion of the SACH foot requires more knee flexion going up, and, if the incline is steep, a shorter prosthetic step. Energy conserving feet provide more dorsiflexion to make this activity easier. Individuals with limited balance and coordination need to be taught each of the advanced activities; more active individuals quickly develop personal techniques after they have learned the basics and have had some practice.

Young clients with long transfemoral residual limbs and good balance and coordination can learn to go down steps one leg over the other by flexing the prosthetic knee on alternate steps. Most will probably be safer using one step at a time. Activities outlined in Tables 9.2 and 9.3 are generally designed for individuals wearing single transfemoral prostheses, but they can be easily adapted for those with one transtibial or another prosthesis. Ambulatory individuals with two transtibial prostheses or one transtibial prosthesis and one transfemoral prosthesis need to adapt the activities. Individuals with two prostheses use a wider base of support and external support such as a cane or crutches. Those with two transtibial prostheses usually lead with the longer

T A B L E   9 . 2   **ADVANCED ACTIVITIES IN THE HOME**

Activity	Procedure
Sitting on the floor	Place the prosthesis about half a step behind the sound foot, keeping the weight on the sound foot. Bend from the waist and flex at the knees and hips, reaching for the floor with both arms outstretched and pivoting to the sound side. Then, gradually lower the body to the floor. This activity is one continuous movement.
Getting up from the floor	Get on hands and knees. Place the sound leg forward, well under the trunk, with the foot flat on the floor while balancing on the hands and the prosthetic knee. Then, extend the sound knee while maintaining the weight over the sound leg. Move to an erect position by pushing strongly with the sound leg and the arms bringing the prosthesis forward when almost erect.
Kneeling	Place the sound foot ahead of the prosthetic foot, keeping the weight on the sound leg. Slowly flex the trunk, hip, and knees until the prosthetic knee can be gently placed on the floor. Clients with transfemoral prostheses can usually kneel on the prosthetic leg, but those with transtibial prostheses find that the patellar bar creates too much pressure in this position. Clients with transtibial prostheses usually kneel on the sound side. Getting up from a kneeling position is like getting up from the floor.
Falling forward	With toes against the mat, pitch forward, breaking the fall with the arms outstretched, thus absorbing the shock with slightly flexed elbows. Partial weight may then be transferred to both knees or rolled onto the unaffected hip, then shoulder.
Falling backward	Flex at the waist so that the buttocks strike the mat first, then roll backward onto the rounded back and shoulders.
Picking up an object from the floor	Place the sound foot ahead of the prosthetic foot with the body weight remaining on the sound leg. Bend forward at the waist, flexing hips and knees until the object can be reached. Care must be taken to maintain weight on the sound leg. Some individuals like to bend sideways rather than forward, while others find it easier to keep the prosthetic knee straight and bend the sound leg until the object can be picked up.

residual limb going up the steps and the shorter coming down (Fig. 9.6). Individuals with one transfemoral prosthesis and one transtibial prosthesis must lead with the transtibial prosthesis going up and with the transfemoral limb coming down. One or two handrails or a handrail and a cane are usually necessary for independent stair climbing. It is unusual for an individual to regain functional ambulation with two transfemoral prostheses because of the amount of energy required. Teaching advanced activities must be individualized according to the type of prostheses, the type of knee control, and the agility of the individual. Those who ambulate with two transfemoral prostheses often have a manual or hydraulic knee lock on one side to provide needed stability for ADL.

OTHER ACTIVITIES

For many people, independent mobility means driving a car. Depending on the side and level of amputation, adjustments to the automobile may or may not be

T A B L E   9 . 3   **ADVANCED ACTIVITIES OUTSIDE THE HOME**

Activity	Procedure
Up and down steps	Lead with the sound foot going up, taking one or two steps at a time. To clear the edge of the step with the prosthesis, extend and slightly abduct the hip and place the prosthetic foot next to the sound foot. Although a handrail may be used for initial practice, full functional rehabilitation requires the ability to go up and down steps without a handrail. Going down, the client leads with the prosthetic foot, making sure the knee is kept locked during weight bearing. The sound leg is brought down on the same step. To go down one leg over the other, place the heel of the prosthetic foot on the edge of the step; shift the weight over the prosthesis, keeping the knee extended. When the sound leg is in position to recover on the next step, flex the prosthetic hip, allowing the knee to buckle, and let the weight go onto the sound leg. Then, extend the prosthetic knee to swing the shin forward over the next lowest step and quickly shift the body weight onto the prosthesis. Continue in a rhythmic progression.
Going up and down inclines	Lead with the sound leg going up inclines, taking a slightly longer step than usual. Hike the prosthetic hip enough to prevent the toe from catching and swing the prosthesis through; avoid abducting it. Take a somewhat shorter step with the prosthetic leg, making sure the knee is extended during weight bearing. The shorter step with the prosthesis compensates for the limited dorsiflexion of the SACH foot. Some trunk flexion may also be needed on very steep hills. Continue up the incline in the line of progression. On very steep hills or for individuals with balance problems, the diagonal method may be more effective. Ascend on the diagonal leading with the sound leg and keeping the prosthetic leg slightly behind the sound leg. On very difficult or slippery inclines, sidestepping, leading with the sound leg, may be the technique of choice. Lead with the prosthetic leg going down an incline, taking a somewhat smaller step than usual and taking particular care to keep the knee extended. Shift weight over the prosthesis and, when the sound foot is in a position to recover, voluntarily flex the prosthetic knee, catching body weight on the sound leg. Modifications include using shorter steps, using repeated single steps, and descending sideways.
Clearing obstacles	Face the obstacle with the sound foot slightly in front and the body weight on the prosthesis. Step over the obstacle with the sound leg, then transfer body weight to the sound leg. Quickly extending the prosthetic hip, forcefully flex the prosthetic hip, whipping the prosthesis forward over the obstacle. Then step forward with a normal gait pattern. An alternate method is to stand sideways to the obstacle with the sound leg closest to the obstacle. With weight on the prosthesis, swing the sound leg over the obstacle and transfer the body weight to the sound leg. Then swing the prosthesis forward, up, and over the obstacle.
Running	Step forward with the sound leg, then shift body weight to the sound leg and hop forward on the sound side. Swing prosthesis forward and shift body weight onto the prosthesis for momentary support. Immediately transfer weight to the sound leg and continue hop-skip running. Some energy conserving or multiaxis feet allow a faster foot flat; slight dorsiflexion in foot alignment allows the amputee to take a longer stride on the sound side. Increased knee friction or a hydraulic unit helps control the swing of the shank during running.

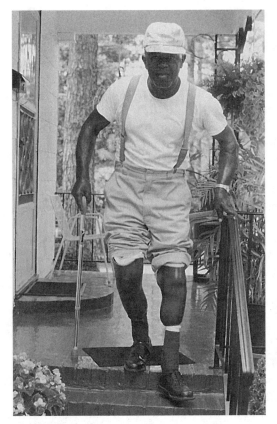

FIGURE 9.6
A client with bilateral transtibial amputations practices going up and down steps.

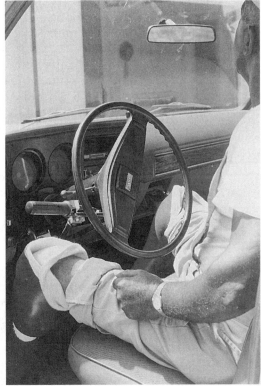

FIGURE 9.7
A client with bilateral transtibial amputations can drive with hand controls.

necessary. For the client with a right-sided amputation, switching the gas or brake pedal for use with the left foot may be necessary. Individuals with bilateral lower extremity amputations need hand controls that allow for operation of the accelerator and brake (Fig. 9.7). Most mechanics can install hand controls or make necessary adaptations to automobiles. Some individuals, particularly those with transfemoral or hip disarticulation amputations, may encounter difficulty getting in and out of the automobile, particularly if it has bucket seats. Two door vehicles fitted with bench seats offer more room for entry and exit. Individuals who have a left prosthesis encounter few problems entering the driver's door, but may have difficulty entering the right passenger door. On the left, they sit in the usual manner and bring the prosthesis in after them. On the right, they need to put the prosthesis in the car first. The situation is reversed for people with a prosthesis on the right. A low steering wheel placement may limit entrance for people with a right transfemoral prosthesis. It is also more difficult to enter the back seat in a two door car.

Public transportation presents hazards, particularly for the elderly and those with multiple amputations. Some individuals are unable to pull themselves up the high first step. In some communities, adapted buses are available. Most clients have no particular problems with trains or airplanes, other than the limited leg room available between seats. The individual with an amputation, particularly at the transfemoral level, may want to choose an aisle seat with the prosthesis close to the aisle. Canes or crutches may be stowed by flight attendants during takeoffs and landings. Individuals who cannot ambulate independently need to make special arrangements with the airlines before any flight.

In some instances, the home needs to be adjusted to make it possible for the person to function independently. Individuals with more than one amputation or those using a wheelchair when not wearing the prosthesis may have difficulty getting in and out of the bathroom or around a two story house. Outside steps without a handrail pose a hazard, particularly in icy weather. Early planning is necessary; a home visit by the therapist can prevent problems later. Elderly individuals may not have the necessary reserve energy for the demands of everyday living with a transfemoral prosthesis and may need to move a bedroom or bathroom to allow them to function on one floor of the home.

Living with a prosthesis also means adjusting to many minor changes in everyday life. The person may not be able to walk as fast as in the past, or may need to alter types of clothing, or learn to cope with the problem of changing shoes. With the prosthesis aligned to one pair of shoes, neither men nor women should wear shoes with different heel heights. This problem is often not mentioned until after the client has been fitted. Many people today wear dress shoes for work, athletic shoes for leisure times, boots in the winter, and sandals in the summer. Each type of shoe has a different heel height and different configuration, but most prosthetic feet do not adapt to different heel heights. The prosthesis is aligned from the ground up and heel height changes are reflected in flexion or extension moments at the knee (see Chap. 8). Sometimes the prosthetic foot can be changed to accommodate various shoes, but this is an expensive procedure. A felt insert in the heel of athletic shoes moderates the problem of the lower heel, but does not solve the problem of shoes with higher heels. Some prosthetic feet do accommodate for different heel heights; the issue needs to be discussed before fitting. Boots restrict ankle movements of the prosthetic foot and sandals are contraindicated for individuals with peripheral vascular disease. Satisfactory adjustment is more likely if the individual is prepared for the many changes that will be required in everyday life.

Recreational Activities

The importance of sport and leisure activities also needs to be considered for the client with an amputation. A full and satisfying lifestyle includes the ability to participate in avocational activities to improve physical fitness, sociability, and self-confidence and just to have fun.

Many activities require little or no adaptation of the prosthesis or of movement patterns. Even those with multiple amputations and those who function primarily with a wheelchair can enjoy playing cards, gardening, or even bowling. More athletically inclined clients can engage in team or individual sports including golf, skiing, swimming, and playing basketball.

Kegal et al.[4] surveyed 100 individuals with unilateral lower extremity amputations to determine their involvement in sports activities. Of the respondents, 60% were active in sports ranging from fishing to jogging. Age, rather than level of amputation, appeared to be the major factor influencing participation. Most returned to sports they performed before their amputations, particularly if the activity did not require running or jumping. Most found it difficult to jog or to go hunting because these activities placed considerable stress on the residual limb. Most respondents wore their regular prosthesis for recreational activities. Seven individuals had special waterproof prostheses, eight used rotation devices in the shank of the prosthesis, and seven used assistive devices, such as crutches or outriggers. Only 28 believed that the prosthetist was knowledgeable about available components for sports. Several had designed their own adaptations. Prosthetists, who were also surveyed, indicated that cost was a major factor in the fabrication of special prostheses for sports, particularly because most third-party payers do not pay for recreational limbs.[3] More recently, Gailey[5] reported on a survey involving 1214 individuals with amputations. The sample was not totally representative because 57% had lost a limb secondary to trauma. However, 60% of respondents stated that they returned to previous activities within 1 year after amputation and 76% indicated they participated in recreational activities including golf, swimming, fishing, and walking. Not all individuals wore their prosthesis for all recreational activities. About 10% reported not wearing the prosthesis at all. Little differences existed between age groups. Although the survey questionnaires were sent to 4000 individuals across the United States, Gailey suggested that more sedentary individuals who had not achieved their desired goals might not have wanted to respond.[5]

During the Vietnam War (1957–1975), the U.S. Army developed a program to teach individuals who had lost limbs how to ski. Those with both unilateral and bilateral amputations learned to ski using one ski and two outriggers. The sports program expanded to include many other activities such as horseback riding, swimming, and even skydiving.[6] Most clients ski on the sound leg with one or two forearm crutches to which a shorter ski foresection has been attached; this is sometimes referred to as three track skiing.[7]

Many people with one prosthesis also continue ballroom dancing, bowling, and weightlifting. Gymnastic activities can be performed by those with two as well as one amputation with little adaptation. Individuals wearing prostheses are able to ice skate and roller skate with little difficulty. The heel height of the prosthetic foot must accommodate the height of the skate shoe, however. Athletic individuals should be encouraged to participate in vigorous physical activities. In too many instances, PTs and PTAs encourage younger clients to pursue exercises and active recreation, but refrain from making similar recommendations to older clients who may well be in greater need of such encouragement.

Outdoor activities, such as camping, fishing, swimming, and water skiing, are also fairly easy to perform with little adaptation. Care should be taken around water to protect the prosthesis from dampness. Most clients swim without a prosthesis; adapted swim fins are useful for individuals with bilateral lower extremity amputations. Hiking and hunting that require walking over uneven ground are stressful on the residual limb. Some individuals use older prostheses with larger sockets and pad the residual limb to reduce torque and rotational stress.

Certain adaptations make participation in sports easier. A rotation component can be installed in the shank of the prosthesis that enables the individual to turn the body as required in golf. Multiaxial and energy conserving feet enhance walking on uneven ground. Many prosthetic feet are designed specifically for running and jumping.[8] Some individuals, particularly those with bilateral lower limb amputations, use adapted wheelchairs.[7]

Highly motivated individuals participate in most sports. Lighter weight components, specially designed knee and foot mechanisms, and well suspended lightweight sockets have increased the competitive abilities of many individuals with amputations. Skilled athletes have successfully participated in competitive sports events all over the world, including the Paraolympics, which are now scheduled the month after the regular Olympics in the same city (Fig. 9.8). Prosthetic manufacturing companies sponsor athletes who help test new components (Fig. 9.9).

Enoka et al.[9] studied the running gait of 10 physically active clients with a unilateral transtibial amputation; 6 were able to run (defined as alternating periods of single support and complete nonsupport in the stride) at speeds ranging from 2.7 to 8.2 meters per second. Three others achieved periods of nonsupport from the intact limb, but not from the prosthesis. Only one individual who had sustained some brain damage was unable to produce nonsupport from either extremity. Marked differences were found in the components of the gait among clients. Over time, each achieved some skill and developed endurance. Light weight, well fitted prostheses with foot mobility were the most advantageous. Running can be a useful sport for people with one transtibial amputation, although more work is needed to develop appropriate prosthetic components.[9] Figure 9.10 depicts the running gait of a person with a transfemoral amputation

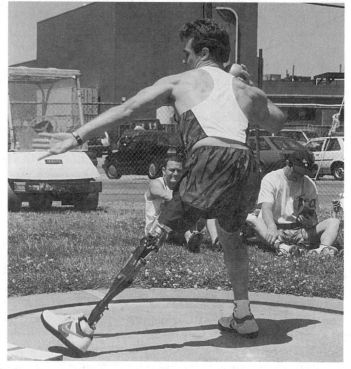

FIGURE 9.8
Mark D'Amico participates in the shotput event in the 1995 National Wheelchair and Amputee Championships. (With permission from Julie M. Gaydos, Orthotic and Prosthetic Athlete Assistance Fund, Inc., and Mark D'Amico.)

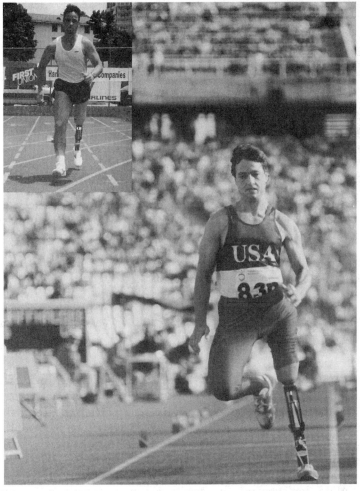

FIGURE 9.9
Todd Schaffhauser uses the Endolite high activity limb in the 1992 Paraolympics in Barcelona. (Courtesy of the Endolite Corporation.)

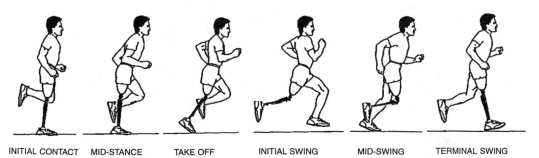

| INITIAL CONTACT | MID-STANCE | TAKE OFF | INITIAL SWING | MID-SWING | TERMINAL SWING |

FIGURE 9.10
Running with a transfemoral prosthesis. (With permission from Gailey, RS, Jr.: Physical therapy management of adult lower limb amputees. In Bowker, JH, and Michael, JW: Atlas of Limb Prosthetics: Surgical, Prosthetic and Rehabilitation Principles, ed 2. Mosby-Yearbook, St Louis, 1992.

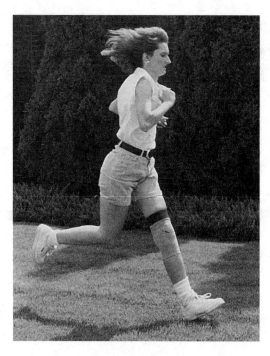

FIGURE 9.11
Running with a transtibial prosthesis.

and a responsive prosthesis. Figure 9.11 depicts an individual running with a transtibial prosthesis.

Individuals with amputations also participate in team sports, although wearing the prosthesis is not always allowed. The National Federation of State High School Associations allows children with lower extremity amputations, particularly transtibial ones, to wear their prostheses while participating in team sports such as football. The rules specify requirements for padding and stipulate that wearing the prosthesis must not place the opponent at a disadvantage. Children with amputations play football, baseball, and volleyball, and even wrestle.[10–12] Individuals with amputations participate in wheelchair basketball. Many have participated in the Wheelchair Olympics. The International Sports Organization for the Disabled classifies handicapped individuals for participation in various sports activities. Leisure and competitive events of all types are available to persons with an amputation.[7,8,11,12] Table 9.4 lists organizations that may be contacted for further information.

Living with an amputation requires physical and emotional adjustments. To a great extent, the fullness of the life of the client is determined by factors that affect most of our lives: family support, financial security, and a healthy body. An amputation does not mitigate against any of these factors, but each person has to develop an individual approach to a satisfying life.

SUMMARY

Rehabilitation of people with one or more amputations is not complete until the person returns to the most fulfilling life possible. Too often, PTs and PTAs set limited ambulatory goals for elderly clients with an amputation and rarely

T A B L E 9 . 4 **RECREATIONAL ASSOCIATIONS FOR HANDICAPPED PERSONS**

American Athletic Association for the Deaf
3607 Washington Blvd., #4
Ogden, UT 84403
(801) 393-8710 (voice); 7916 (TTY)

Dwarf Athletic Association of America
418 Willow Way
Lewisville, TX 75067
(214) 317-8299

Adapted Sports Association, Inc.
University of Toledo
2801 West Bancroft St.
Toledo, OH 43606

Adaptive Sports Program
6832 Marlette Road
Marlette, MI 48453

Aircraft Hands Control
Ed Stakleman
P.O. Box 207
Sturgis, KY 42459

American Amputee Foundation
Box 55218, Hillcrest Station
Little Rock, AR 72225

American Alliance for Health, Physical
   Education, and Recreation
1201 Sixteenth St., NW
Washington, DC 20036

American Camping Association
Bradford Woods
Martinsville, Indiana 46151

American Water Ski Association
P.O. Box 191
Winter Haven, FL 33880

American Wheelchair Bowling Association
N54W15858
Menomonee Falls, WI 53051

American Wheelchair Pilots Association
4419 North 27th St.
Phoenix, AZ 85016

Amputee Golfers Association
Box 1228
Amherst, NH 03031
(800) 633-NAGA

Amputees in Motion
Box 2703
Escondido, CA 92025

Amputee Soccer International
c/o Johnson and Higgins
1215 Fourth Ave
Seattle, WA 98161

Disabled Sportsmen of America, Inc.
P.O. Box 26
Vinton, VA 24179

International WC Road Racers
30 Myano Lane, Box 3
Stamford, CT 06902

National Handicapped Sports
451 Hungerford Dr., Suite 100
Rockville, MD 20850
(301) 217-0960

Handicapped SCUBA Association
116 West El Portal, Suite 104
San Clemente, CA 92672

National Wheelchair Athletic Association
3595 East Fountain Blvd., Suite L-1
Colorado Springs, CO 80910

International Sports Organization for the Disabled
1600 James Naismith Drive
Gloucester, Ontario, K1B 5N4
Canada

US Association of Blind Athletes
33 North Institute St.
Colorado Springs, CO 80903
(719) 630-0422

US Cerebral Palsy Athletic Association
3810 W. Northwest Highway, #205
Dallas, TX 75220
(214) 351-1510

US Les Autres Sports Assoc
1475 W. Gray, Suite 166
Houston, TX 77019
(713) 521-3737

Wheelchair Sports USA
3595 E. Fountain Blvd., #L-1
Colorado Springs, CO 80910
(719) 574-1150

US Wheelchair Racquet Sports Association
1941 Viento Verano Drive
Diamond Bar, CA 91765

US Amputee Athletic Association
Box 560686
Charlotte, NC 28256

inform the person of the potential for participation in a full array of activities. Current reimbursement policies negatively affect the ability to help the individual develop competence in advanced activities. If full training is not possible, teaching basic and advanced activities needs to be a part of the total rehabilitation programs, along with exposure to the potential for recreational pursuits. Long-term follow-up is also necessary to ensure the continued function of appliances and to prevent complications.

REFERENCES

1. MacBride, A, Rogers, J, Whylie, B, and Freeman, SJ: Psychosocial factors in the rehabilitation of elderly amputees. Psychosomatics 21:258–265, 1980.
2. Comfort A: Sexual Consequences of Disability, George F Stickley, Philadelphia, 1978.
3. English, RD, Hubbard, WA, and McElroy, GK: Establishment of consistent gait after fitting new components. J Rehabil Res Dev 32:32–35, 1995.
4. Kegel, B, Webster, JC, and Burgess, EM: Recreational activities of lower extremity amputees: A survey. Arch Phys Med Rehabil 61:258–264, 1980.
5. Gailey, RS, Jr: Recreational pursuits for elders with amputation. Topics in Geriatric Rehabilitation 8:39–58, 1992.
6. Smith, JP: In what sports can patients with amputations and other handicaps successfully and actively participate? Phys Ther 50:121–126, 1970.
7. Kegel, B: Adaptations for sports and recreation. In Bowker, JH, and Michael, JW (eds.): Atlas of Limb Prosthetics: Surgical, Prosthetic, and Rehabilitation Principles, ed. 2. Mosby-Year Book, St. Louis, 1992, pp. 623–654.
8. Mensch, G, and Ellis, PM: Physical Therapy Management of Lower Extremity Amputations. Aspen Publishers, Rockville, MD, 1986.
9. Enoka, RM, Miller, DI, and Burgess, EM: Below-knee amputee running gait. Am J Phys Med 61:66–84, 1982.
10. Adams, RC, Daniel, AN, McCubbin, JA, and Rullman, L: Games, Sports and Exercises for the Physically Handicapped, ed. 3. Lea & Febiger, Philadelphia, 1982.
11. Dodds, JW: Sports and amputees. In Karacoloff, LA, Hammersley, CS, and Schneider, FJ: Lower Extremity Amputation: A Guide to Functional Outcomes in Physical Therapy Management, ed. 2. Aspen Publishers, Gaithersburg, MD, 1992, pp. 183–196.
12. Burgess, EM, and Rappoport, A: Physical Fitness: A Guide for Individuals with Lower Limb Loss. Department of Veterans Affairs; Veterans Health Administration, Washington, DC, 1992.

chapter ten

Upper Limb Amputations

Joan Edelstein

OBJECTIVES

At the end of this chapter, all students are expected to:

1   List the etiologies for upper limb amputation.

2   Describe upper limb amputation surgery.

3   Outline a program for postsurgical management.

4   Compare the prosthetic replacements for the human hand.

5   Indicate the components of the most common transradial (below elbow) prostheses.

6   Develop a training program for a client fitted with a unilateral transradial prosthesis.

Upper limb amputation is much less common than lower limb amputation. Consequently, physical therapists (PTs), physical therapist assistants (PTAs), and other clinicians are unlikely to acquire substantial experience with such clients, unless employed in a specialized rehabilitation center. Nevertheless, it is important to recognize the basic elements of surgical and postoperative care, as well as the extent of contemporary prosthetic replacement, so that the clinician is prepared to treat the occasional client. The purpose of this chapter is to introduce PTs to major considerations in management of clients with upper limb loss. Although amputation occurs at every level, from loss of a phalanx to loss of the entire limb, prosthetic use is most likely among individuals with transradial (below elbow) amputation.[1-3] Consequently, this chapter focuses on rehabilitation of a client who will ultimately be fitted with a transradial prosthesis. Many treatment principles already described for clients with lower limb amputation also apply to individuals with loss of the upper limb.

case study

George Wilson, a 22-year-old carpenter's apprentice, sustained traumatic transradial amputation of his right hand while at work. He was referred to physical therapy 2 days after surgical revision of the wound.

CASE STUDY ACTIVITIES

1 What are the most pertinent elements in evaluating this client?
2 What are the client's likely psychological responses?
3 What measures will foster optimal independence in daily activities?
4 How should Mr. Wilson be prepared for prosthetic fitting?

Surgery

By far, the most typical client with upper limb amputation is a young man who has sustained trauma.[4] Although improvements in microsurgery occasionally enable limb reattachment, normal motor and sensory function are seldom restored. Other common causes are congenital limb anomaly and bone tumor. Most clients are children or young adults who heal rapidly. Postsurgically, the limb may be encased in a rigid plaster of paris dressing or simply in sterile gauze. The plaster cast prevents edema formation, thus reducing postoperative pain and hastening healing.[5] The cast also serves as the foundation for a prosthesis to enable the client to grasp objects soon after surgery; such usage is associated with greater likelihood of eventual acceptance of a permanent prosthesis.[6] Although the gauze dressing is easier to remove for wound inspection, it neither controls edema nor permits attachment of a temporary prosthesis. Most children with congenital limb absence do not require surgical revision. Clients with tumors may be treated with a combination of surgery and radiation. The level of amputation is determined by the site and extent of the tumor.

Postsurgical Management

The goals of postsurgical management are to:

1 Achieve wound healing.
2 Reduce pain.
3 Maintain mobility of all proximal joints.
4 Maintain motor power at all proximal joints.
5 Enable the client to achieve maximum independence in daily activities.
6 Address the emotional aspects of amputation.

Evaluation

Evaluation of the new client includes measurement of limb length. The length designations are related to prosthetic components and residual anatomic function. For transradial amputation, a tape measure is stretched from the medial humeral epicondyle to the ulnar styloid on the sound side. On the amputated side, the landmarks are the medial epicondyle to the end of the more distal forearm bone; if the client has excessive soft tissue at the end of the limb, the tissue should be compressed to obtain an accurate measurement. Using these two measurements, the therapist computes the percentage of limb loss. The standard measurements and nomenclature[7] for limb length are:

100%	Wrist disarticulation
100% to 55%	Long transradial
55% to 35%	Short transradial
35% to 0%	Very short transradial

For transhumeral amputation, a tape measure is stretched from the acromion to the lateral humeral epicondyle on the sound side. On the amputated side, the landmarks are the acromion to the end of the humerus. Transhumeral percentages and nomenclature are:

90% to 100%	Elbow disarticulation
50% to 90%	Standard transhumeral
30% to 50%	Short transhumeral
0% to 30%	Humeral neck
0%	Shoulder disarticulation

Absence of any portion of thorax or shoulder girdle is termed a **forequarter amputation.**

Range of motion is also measured at all proximal joints. The client who is to be fitted with a prosthesis operated by a harness and cable needs ample mobility of the shoulder and shoulder girdle. Regardless of the type of prosthesis, the client should have full range of elbow motion to facilitate grooming. Forearm motion is reduced when the interosseous membrane between the radius and ulna becomes fibrotic. Reduced mobility limits the client's active pronation and supination. The prosthesis has a component that provides forearm motion; however, the more active motion that is retained, the less the client will need to rely on a mechanism. Individuals with short and very short transradial amputations retain virtually no pronation and supination. Although wrist disarticulation preserves the distal radioulnar joint, the client usually has diminished forearm rotation. Lacking a hand, the person has little need to pronate and supinate. In addition, the postsurgical dressing may force the forearm bones together, thus fostering contracture. The most effective way to reduce contracture is to encase the forearm in a plaster dressing that is shaped to emphasize separation of the bones.

Clients with short and very short transradial amputations are apt to have limited elbow excursion. A manual muscle test is a basic part of evaluation, as is skin inspection. The therapist should also note the client's general cognitive status and emotional response to the amputation. Other elements to be evaluated include determining the dominant arm before amputation and the condition of the scar and the skin on the amputated limb and shoulder.

For individuals with transhumeral amputations, the treatment plan includes exercise to maintain maximum mobility of the shoulder and shoulder girdle.

Most amputation wounds heal readily, particularly if the client has a rigid dressing. Postoperative pain may be localized to the operative site, phantom, or both. Local pain often indicates infection that may require debridement and appropriate medication. Like the client with lower limb amputation, the client with upper limb amputation is likely to feel that the missing body part is still present. When the feeling is not painful, the phenomenon is termed **phantom sensation.** The client should be reassured that this experience is normal, given the large cerebral representation of the hand. When the client complains of burning, throbbing, electrical shocks, or other unpleasant sensations, the phenomenon is termed **phantom pain.** Although no treatment eradicates phantom pain for all clients, the wide repertory of available approaches should include at least one that will be effective for any given client (see Chap. 5). Some clients respond to bilateral exercise, in which the individual flexes and extends the fingers on the sound hand against resistance while imagining that the absent hand is also exercising. One might also use ultrasound, transcutaneous electrical neural stimulation (TENS), massage, or functional activity. Massage is especially useful to help the client gain tolerance to the pressure that will be applied by the prosthetic socket, as well as to prevent adhesions.

Most clients retain adequate motor power unless the trauma that caused the amputation also injured nerves or tendons or caused excessive scar tissue. The client should have a program of maintenance exercises that emphasize isometric contraction of the forearm flexors and extensors, if myoelectric fitting is contemplated. For those who will probably have a prosthesis with cable and harness control, emphasis is on strength in the shoulder and shoulder girdle. Restoring functional activities is an excellent way to promote motor power and joint mobility. As soon as the wound heals, the client should be encouraged to resume self care, especially personal hygiene, dressing, feeding, writing, and similar activities. For some activities, for example, buttoning a shirt, the client will find it easier to use the sound hand, even if that hand was not the dominant one before the amputation. The sound hand retains dexterity and sensation. Because approximately half of those with upper limb amputation lose the dominant hand, an important element in early management is teaching change of dominance. Although the client may decide to write with the prosthesis eventually, other activities are generally easier with the intact hand. The client may experience an initial period of clumsiness and frustration, but with the PT's encouragement and support should retain or gain considerable independence with the sound hand.

PTs and all members of the rehabilitation team should not underestimate the emotional impact of upper limb amputation. Unlike lower limb amputation that usually follows several years of increasing disability caused by peripheral vascular disease, most arm amputations occur accidentally on the job or during recreation. For most people, the hand has much more psychological importance than the foot. One holds a child's hand and strokes a loved one's brow with a hand. Loss of the hand cannot be disguised effectively. The rehabilitation team must deeply empathize with the client's loss, calmly accept the humanity of the individual whether or not both hands are present, and perceptively guide the client to the realization that he or she can lead a fully satisfying work and social life even with upper limb loss. Exploring the client's goals for rehabilitation helps clinical team members to comprehend the degree of understanding and acceptance that the client possesses. Psychosocial support is critical to fostering a positive rehabilitation outcome; a psychologist, social worker, or counselor can help the client cope with the emotional effects of the amputation.

Prosthetic Replacement

c a s e s t u d y

Mr. Wilson's wound has healed. He has learned to tolerate the sensation of the missing right hand. He has excellent motor power throughout the upper limb, as well as full range of motion in the shoulder and elbow. Because the amputation occurred through the middle third of the forearm, pronation and supination are limited. He can now bathe; attend to toilet activities; and groom, dress, and feed himself independently. He still has difficulty writing rapidly with his left hand. He is aware that several types of prostheses are available and is eager to be fitted.

CASE STUDY ACTIVITIES

1 Compare the passive hand, cable controlled hand, myoelectric hand, and hook with regard to appearance, function, weight, cost, and durability. Which is most suitable for Mr. Wilson? Why?

2 What are the proximal components of the below-elbow prosthesis?

Lower limb amputation affects the individual's lifestyle profoundly, compelling some provision for locomotion, whether with a prosthesis or a wheelchair. In contrast, upper limb amputation has much less effect on performance of daily activities and many vocational and recreational pursuits. Consequently, many clients with unilateral upper limb amputation elect not to wear a prosthesis. They find ways of accomplishing activities or of foregoing those that no longer seem important, preferring to avoid problems of prosthetic discomfort, maintenance, and cost. Most individuals with transradial amputation, however, do find a prosthesis worthwhile.[1–2]

Prosthetic Replacements for the Hand

Of paramount importance to the client and the rehabilitation team is the prosthetic component that will substitute for the missing hand. No device completely replaces the appearance or function of the anatomic hand. Nevertheless, the prosthetic counterpart, called a **terminal device,** can contribute to the wearer's function and self-esteem. The two types of terminal device are the hand and the hook. Either is secured to a plastic socket encasing the forearm. Table 10.1 provides a comparison of terminal devices.

PROSTHETIC HANDS

Most adult clients, or the parents of children with amputations, are keenly interested in replacing the lost hand with a terminal device that resembles a hand (Fig. 10.1).[3,9] Two groups of such components are manufactured: (1) passive hands that have no moving parts; and (2) active hands that have a mechanism that permits the client to control finger position by appropriate action in the proximal part of the amputated limb. Both active and passive hands are made in a range of sizes to suit most children and adults. Both are covered with a flexible plastic glove that matches the client's skin tone. Many people enhance the hand's appearance by wearing a ring or other jewelry on it. The glove will

T A B L E 1 0 . 1 **COMPARISON OF TERMINAL DEVICES**

Component	Appearance	Function	Weight for Adult Size
Passive hand	Anthropomorphic shape. Sizes to suit 1½-year-old child to medium-sized man. Glove similar to wearer's skin color.	Can stabilize objects on a table. Wearer can adjust finger position passively.	8 oz. with glove.
Cable operated hand	Same as above.	Wearer can adjust finger position by shoulder motion that causes tension in the control cable in the hand.	14 oz. with glove.
Myoelectric hand	Same as previous	Wearer can adjust finger position by contracting forearm muscles that activate motor in the hand.	22 oz. with glove and battery.
Cable operated hook	Shiny metal tool. Child-size hooks available with pink or brown plastic coating.	Wearer can adjust finger position by shoulder motion that causes tension in the control cable on the hook.	3 oz.

stain and tear and should be replaced at least once a year to retain optimal appearance.

Compared with active hands, passive hands are lighter, less expensive, and more durable. The fingers are made of a flexible wire covered with resilient

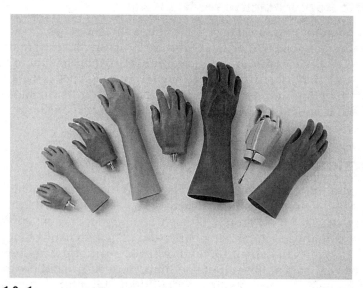

FIGURE 10.1
Prosthetic hands and gloves in child, adolescent, and adult sizes. (Courtesy of Hosmer Dorrance Corp., Campbell, CA.)

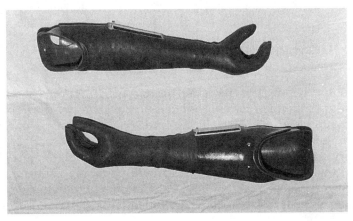

FIGURE 10.2
Myoelectric transradial prosthesis with hand and cosmetic glove.

plastic. The wearer can bend or straighten the fingers with the sound hand. Clients use the passive hand not only to restore normal appearance, but also to assist in such tasks as holding a large package and to stabilize paper while writing with the other hand. The passive hand, however, has no grasp function.

Active hands do enable grasping. Commercially available hands have a mechanism that moves the thumb, index, and middle fingers; the fourth and fifth fingers remain passive. The prehension pattern is a three jaw chuck that permits the wearer to hold many common objects securely. The hands do not open as widely as the anatomic hand; consequently, the client can grasp only things that have a cross section smaller than 10 centimeters (about 4 inches).

The most popular active hand is operated myoelectrically[9] (Fig. 10.2). The client wears a socket that has one or more skin electrodes that contact appropriate muscle groups. When the client contracts the muscle, the electrode transmits the microvoltage generated by the muscle to a mechanism that causes the electrical signal to operate a small motor that, in turn, enables the hand mechanism to open or close the fingers. The motor is powered by a battery worn inside the prosthetic socket or, in the case of wrist disarticulation, elsewhere on the client's body. Myoelectric control can provide excellent grasp force. Adept users control finger opening and closing easily, although some clients may require many months to gain proficiency.[10]

The other type of prosthetic hand has a steel cable that is attached to a trunk harness. By flexing the shoulder, the client puts tension on the cable that pulls on the hand mechanism and causes the fingers either to open (voluntary opening) or to close (voluntary closing).[9] Relaxing tension on the cable allows the fingers to revert to the opposite position. Thus, in a voluntary opening device, relaxation causes the fingers to close. Grasp force in the voluntary opening device is determined by springs in the mechanism and is comparatively weak. Grasp force in the voluntary closing device is determined by the force that the client applies to the cable; consequently, the user can achieve substantial force. Although lighter and less expensive than myoelectric hands, cable operated devices require the client to wear a harness that some find intrusive. The harness also tends to restrict the work space in which the client can use the prostheses easily.[11]

HOOKS

A hook (Fig. 10.3) is the other basic type of terminal device. Made either of aluminum or steel, mass produced hooks have two fingers that the client can open and close. Myoelectrically controlled hooks are manufactured; however, most clients who wear hooks have cable operated models that are either voluntary opening or voluntary closing. The most common hook is voluntary opening, in which grasp force is determined by rubber bands encircling the base of the fingers. Cable operated hooks are much lighter than any other type of device and are less expensive. Hooks are also more durable. Because the tips of the

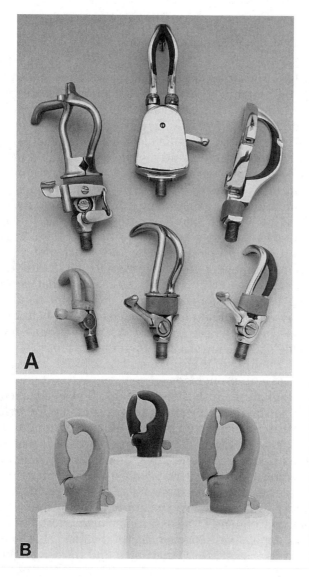

FIGURE 10.3
Hook terminal devices. (*A*) Top left: voluntary opening hook with locking mechanism; top middle: voluntary closing hook; top right: voluntary closing hook; bottom left: infant size voluntary opening hook; bottom middle: adult size voluntary opening hook; bottom right: adolescent size voluntary opening hook. (Courtesy of Hosmer Dorrance Corp., Campbell, CA.) (*B*) Voluntary closing aluminum, steel, and polyurethane terminal devices; left: tan plastic, adolescent size; middle: dark brown child size; right: tan adult size. (Courtesy of TRS Inc., Boulder, CO.)

fingers of the hook are relatively small, the client can see the object to be grasped more easily than with the thicker fingers of a prosthetic hand.[12]

TERMINAL DEVICE SELECTION

No terminal device truly replaces a lost hand; consequently, the rehabilitation team and the client must determine the best compromise on an individual basis. Although some clients are provided with two or more terminal devices in an attempt to increase functional restoration, most individuals find that one device serves adequately and rarely use the other device. The team and client must assess the relative importance of appearance, amount of grasp power needed, economy, durability, and prosthetic weight to arrive at a reasoned prescription. See Table 10.2 for a comparison of cost and durability. Vocational and social pursuits are major determinants in the choice of terminal device. For example, the individual whose job involves use of tools and abrasive materials will find that a hook, being more durable, is an appropriate choice. The client with a very short transradial amputation may become fatigued after repeatedly lifting the relatively heavier myoelectric hand. Someone who has a desk job probably will prefer a hand. Although a hook is conspicuously different from a hand, people who use a hook proficiently are usually able to return to the community without much embarrassment.

Prosthetic Replacements for the Wrist and Forearm

The hand, of whatever design, is secured to a wrist unit. In most instances, the wrist unit does not replace the functions of the anatomic wrist, namely dorsiflexion, palmar flexion, and ulnar and radial deviation. Instead, the wrist unit replaces forearm motion and permits the client to pronate and supinate the terminal device. For individuals with high bilateral amputations, a prosthesis

T A B L E   1 0 . 2   **COST AND DURABILITY OF TERMINAL DEVICES**

Component	Cost	Durability
Passive hand	Moderately expensive	Glove is vulnerable to stains and tears.
Cable operated hand	Moderately expensive, more expensive than passive hand.	Glove is vulnerable to stains and tears. Mechanism may malfunction. Fingers or cable may break when moderate force applied.
Myoelectric hand	Most expensive	Glove is vulnerable to stains and tears. Battery requires periodic recharging and eventual replacement. Mechanism and especially its electrical components may malfunction. Fingers may break when moderate force is applied.
Cable operated hook	Least expensive	Rubber lining is vulnerable to abrasion. Fingers or cable may break when extreme force is applied.

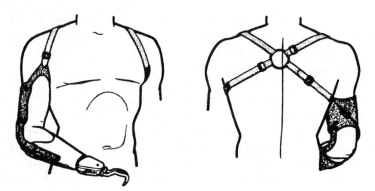

FIGURE 10.4
Figure of eight harness for a transradial prosthesis with tricep pad and hook.

may be fitted with a wrist unit that allows palmar flexion as well as pronation and supination (flexion unit). The flexion unit enables the wearer to reach the midline of the body, which is important for eating, buttoning, and toilet activities.

PROXIMAL PARTS OF TRANSRADIAL PROSTHESES

The wrist unit is embedded in the distal end of the socket. Sockets are custom made plastic fittings intended to fit snugly to distribute pressure over the largest area. The proximal portion of the transradial socket terminates in the vicinity of the humeral epicondyles. A self suspending socket supports the weight of the terminal device and wrist unit by a secure hold at the epicondyles, thus eliminating the need for harness suspension. Self suspending sockets are often used with myoelectric hands.

A harness is necessary to suspend a socket that is not supported by the epicondyles, to transmit shoulder motions to a cable, or for both functions. The harness is made of dacron or a fiber blend webbing (Fig. 10.4). The customary design, figure of eight, has a loop around each shoulder; these loops connect in back. One strap from the loop on the amputated side is buckled to the cable that controls the terminal device. The other strap from the loop on the amputated side is buckled to an inverted Y strap that lies on the anterior surface of the upper arm and suspends the prosthesis. The loop on the sound side is termed the **axillary loop.**

PROXIMAL PARTS OF TRANSHUMERAL PROSTHESES

The prosthesis for the individual whose amputation is at the level of elbow disarticulation or higher includes a terminal device, a wrist unit, a forearm shell to replace the length of the absent forearm, an elbow unit, a socket, and a suspension (Fig. 10.5). All elbow units have a hinge for elbow flexion and a locking mechanism to enable to wearer to retain the desired flexion angle. For the client whose amputation is at the standard transhumeral level or higher, the elbow unit also incorporates a turntable that allows the individual to rotate the forearm

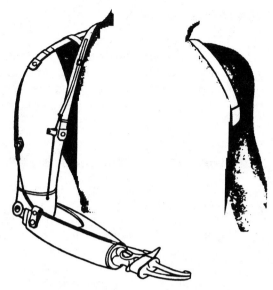

FIGURE 10.5
Transhumeral prosthesis with figure of eight harness.

shell medially and laterally. The elbow unit connects the forearm shell with the socket. A harness, typically a transhumeral figure of eight, suspends the prosthesis and transmits motions of the shoulder and shoulder girdle to the cable system. Ordinarily, one cable operates the terminal device and the elbow hinge, whereas a second cable operates the elbow lock.

Prosthetic Training

The elements of upper limb prosthetic training are donning and doffing, use of controls, use in bimanual function, and learning or relearning vocational skills. Careful evaluation of prosthetic fit and function of all components should precede training.[13]

DONNING AND DOFFING

Regardless of the type of prosthesis, the client must be able to don it independently. Otherwise, the individual is almost certain to abandon wearing it after discharge from the rehabilitation center. Donning a prosthesis that has a figure of eight harness involves (1) applying a cotton or wool sock; (2) inserting the residual limb in the socket; and finally (3) inserting the sound limb through the axillary loop. To doff the prosthesis, the client reverses the steps, that is, removes the axillary loop, withdraws the residual limb from the socket, and removes the sock.

To don a myoelectrically controlled transradial prosthesis, the client (1) dons a cotton stockinette tube, taking care that the proximal margin of the stockinette is above the antecubital fossa; (2) applies the socket; and (3) pulls the distal end of the stockinette through a hole in the socket, thereby drawing the superficial tissue of the forearm snugly into the socket. The client thus does not wear a sock. Ordinarily, the prosthesis has no harness. Doffing involves twisting the socket to loosen it from the epicondyles and distal tissue.

CONTROLS TRAINING

Teaching controls usage encompasses every element the client requires to operate the prosthesis correctly. The transradial prosthesis has only two components that the client must control, the terminal device and the wrist unit. Although the transhumeral prosthesis is more complex, the basic principles of controls training for a transradial prosthesis remain valid.[13]

TERMINAL DEVICE TRAINING: MYOELECTRIC

Before the prosthesis is made, the client undergoes preliminary training to determine the best site for electrode placement.[14] The therapist uses a surface electrode and a voltmeter to explore the forearm for sites where the client can produce the greatest electrical response. Most myoelectric systems have one electrode on the flexors and another on the extensors. Thus, preliminary training is devoted to locating optimal sites and to guiding the client to contract one muscle group isometrically while maintaining relaxation of its antagonists. When the sites have been identified, the client practices with a test socket that has electrodes. The test socket facilitates alteration in electrode positioning. After final electrode positions have been determined, the prosthetist fabricates the permanent socket with incorporated electrodes. With this permanent socket, the client practices contraction of the flexors to close the hand and contraction of the extensors to open the hand. The goal is accurate hand function without unwanted finger motion. The client concentrates on the movement of the hand by watching the way the fingers move; eventually the person develops proprioceptive appreciation of the amount of muscular activity necessary to produce the desired amount of finger motion.

TERMINAL DEVICE TRAINING: CABLE OPERATED

The therapist instructs the client to flex the shoulder to operate the terminal device, whether voluntary opening or voluntary closing. Initially, the elbow should be flexed 90 degrees so that the client can see the terminal device easily and so that cable alignment is optimal. Sometimes it is necessary to resist shoulder flexion so that the client can put sufficient tension on the cable to affect the terminal device. After the client realizes the relation of shoulder flexion to terminal device operation, training is devoted to refining control motions.

The client should keep the contralateral, or sound, arm relaxed. Training helps the client recognize that the same body motion is effective regardless of the position of the elbow and shoulder. The therapist then places the terminal device close to the client's chest and asks the client to operate the device. Scapular abduction is necessary because shoulder flexion would cause the terminal device to move away from the chest.

With a voluntary opening terminal device, the client should practice maintaining slight tension on the control cable to prevent the hand or hook fingers from closing completely; this skill is used when handling fragile objects (Fig. 10.6). With a voluntary closing terminal device, the client should practice applying the gentle tension on the control cable that will be necessary when dealing with objects that might crush or tear (Fig. 10.7).

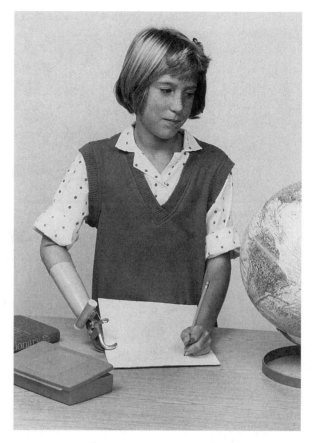

FIGURE 10.6
Child using a transradial prosthesis with electrically controlled voluntary opening hook. (Courtesy of Hosmer Dorrance Corp., Campbell, CA.)

WRIST UNIT

Most wrist units are passive; that is, the client changes the position of the unit by turning the terminal device with the sound hand, or nudges the terminal device against the edge of a table or the chest, thigh, or contralateral forearm. If the wrist unit has a locking mechanism, the therapist teaches the client how

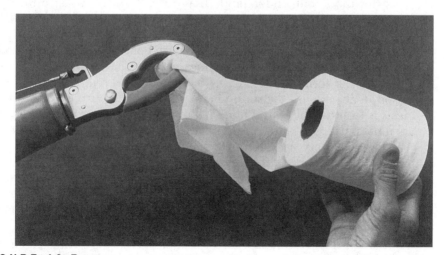

FIGURE 10.7
Grasping toilet tissue with voluntary closing terminal device. (Courtesy of TRS Inc., Boulder, CO.)

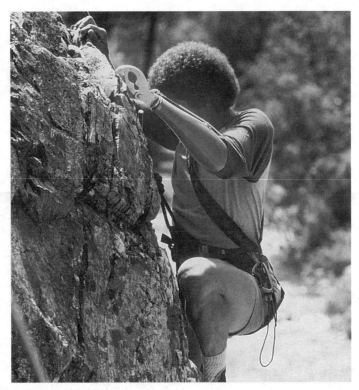

FIGURE 10.8
Adult using a transradial prosthesis with voluntary closing terminal device to aid in mountain climbing. (Courtesy of TRS Inc., Boulder, CO.)

to lock and unlock it by means of a lever or rotating rings on the unit. If the wrist unit is controlled by a cable or by myoelectric mechanism, the therapist teaches the client the correct sequence of motions to effect change in terminal device position.

After the client understands how to control the wrist unit, the therapist introduces a form board to help the individual integrate terminal device and wrist unit operation. The form board consists of objects of various sizes, shapes, textures, and weights. The purpose of form board training is to increase skill in use of the prosthesis. The client does not use the sound hand. Of course, the artificiality of form board training is evident; in a real life situation, the client grasps an object with the sound hand. Because the purpose of a unilateral pros-thesis is to assist the sound hand in complex maneuvers, however, the individ-ual must be able to control the prosthesis independently (Fig. 10.8).

It is relatively easy to grasp a hard rubber cube; the client pronates the terminal device, opens it so that the finger tips are slightly farther apart than the width of the cube, then closes it (or allows the fingers to close). It is more difficult to manage a thin metal disc. The client will find that placing the ter-minal device in midposition between pronation and supination affords the best approach to the disc. Any object that is easy to deform, such as a paper cup or a foam rubber ball, requires the client to maintain tension on the control cable with a voluntary opening terminal device, or to apply minimum tension on the control cable with a voluntary closing device, or to contract forearm flexors gently with a myoelectrically controlled device.

FUNCTIONAL USE TRAINING

In this next step in rehabilitation, the client is guided to use the prosthesis to assist the sound hand in the performance of bimanual activities. Because most daily tasks can be accomplished with a single hand, the therapist must be creative in selecting those that are easier to execute bimanually. The basic principle is that the prosthesis performs the more static part of the task. For example, when cutting meat with a knife and fork, one stabilizes the meat with the fork held in the prosthesis while using the knife with the sound hand. Some other bimanual activities are opening and applying an adhesive bandage, hammering nails, pulling on socks, folding a letter and inserting it in an envelope, and wrapping a package. (Some tasks, such as tying shoelaces, can be done either with one hand or with a prosthesis.)[15]

VOCATIONAL TRAINING

Because most people who sustain upper limb amputation are men of working age, it is important to explore vocations that can be pursued with or without a prosthesis. Preparing to return to work is a great motivator for many people. Few jobs are beyond the capability of people with upper limb amputation. Although the rehabilitation program is generally not designed to include specific job training, the clinical team should conduct prevocational exploration, vocational assessment, or refer the client to a job training center.

SUMMARY

Upper limb amputation is relatively unusual. The most common cause is trauma, particularly affecting young men. Surgical management may include use of a rigid postoperative dressing. Postsurgically, the therapist is concerned with wound healing, pain reduction, maintaining joint mobility and motor power, and the client's resumption of independent daily activities. The team also addresses the emotional impact of amputation. The transradial prosthesis consists of a terminal device, either a hand or a hook; a wrist unit; and a socket; if the terminal device is cable operated, the prosthesis also has a harness. The steps in education are donning, controls training, functional use training, and vocational training.

GLOSSARY

Cable	The metal cord that connects the harness to the terminal device and transmits the power to the terminal device from shoulder motion.
Hook	A type of terminal device that has two metal fingers.
Myoelectric	Type of control using muscle contraction to provide an electrical current to a terminal device.

Terminal device	Part of the prosthesis that replaces the hand. The terminal device may be an artificial hand or a hook.
Test socket	A preliminary socket constructed to ensure proper fit and power attachments.
Voluntary closing	A terminal device that closes with muscle movement and opens with relaxation.
Voluntary opening	A terminal device that opens with muscle movement and closes with relaxation.

REFERENCES

1. Millstein, SG, Heger, H, and Hunter, GA: Prosthetic use in adult upper limb amputees: A comparison of the body powered and electrically powered prostheses. Prosthetics and Orthotics International 10:2734, 1986.
2. Sturup, J, Thyregod, HC, Jensen, JS, et al: Traumatic amputation of the upper limb: The use of body-powered prostheses and employment consequences. Prosthetics and Orthotics International 12:50–52, 1988.
3. Van Lunteren, A, Van Lunteren-Gerritsen, GHM, Stassen, HG, and Zuithoff, MJ: A field evaluation of arm prostheses for unilateral amputees. Prosthetics and Orthotics International 7:141–151, 1983.
4. Ouellette, EA: Wrist disarticulation and transradial amputation: Surgical principles. In Bowker, JH, and Michael, JW (eds.): Atlas of Limb Prosthetics: Surgical, Prosthetic, and Rehabilitation Principles, ed. 2. Mosby-Year Book, St. Louis, 1992, pp. 237–240.
5. Malone, JM, Fleming, LL, Robertson, J, et al: Immediate, early, and late postsurgical management of upper-limb amputation. J Rehabil Res Dev 21:33–41, 1984.
6. Brenner, CD: Wrist disarticulation and transradial amputation: Prosthetic principles. In Bowker, JH, and Michael, JW (eds.): Atlas of Limb Prosthetics: Surgical, Prosthetic, and Rehabilitation Principles, ed. 2. Mosby-Year Book, St. Louis, 1992, pp. 241–250.
7. Muilenberg, AL, and LeBlanc, MA: Body-powered upper-limb components. In Atkins, DJ, and Meier RH (eds.): Comprehensive Management of the Upper-Limb Amputee, Springer, New York, 1989, pp. 29–38.
8. Atkins, DJ: Postoperative and preprosthetic therapy programs. In Atkins, DJ, and Meier, RH (eds.): Comprehensive Management of the Upper-Limb Amputee. Springer, New York, 1989, pp. 11–18.
9. Billock, JN: Upper limb prosthetic terminal devices: Hands versus hooks. Clin Prosthet Orthot 10:57–65, 1986.
10. Edelstein, JE, and Berger, N: Performance comparison among children fitted with myoelectric and body-powered hands. Arch Phys Med Rehabil 74:376–380, 1993.
11. Stein, RB, and Walley, M: Functional comparison of upper extremity amputees using myoelectric and conventional prostheses. Arch Phys Med Rehabil 64:243–248, 1983.
12. Murphy, EF: In support of the hook. Clin Prosthet Orthot 10:78–81, 1986.
13. Atkins, DJ: Adult upper-limb prosthetic training. In Atkins, DJ, and Meier, RH (eds.): Comprehensive Management of the Upper-Limb Amputee. Springer, New York, 1989, pp. 39–59.
14. Spiegel, SR: Adult myoelectric upper-limb prosthetic training. In Atkins, DJ, and Meier, RH (eds.): Comprehensive Management of the Upper-Limb Amputee. Springer, New York, 1989, pp. 60–71.
15. Edelstein, JE: Special considerations: Rehabilitation without prostheses: Functional skills training. In Bowker, JH, and Michael JW (eds.): Atlas of Limb Prosthetics: Surgical, Prosthetic, and Rehabilitation Principles, ed. 2. Mosby-Year Book, St. Louis, 1992, pp. 721–728.

chapter eleven

The Child with an Amputation

OBJECTIVES

At the end of this chapter, all students are expected to:

1   Classify congenital amputations according to standard terminology.

2   Differentiate between congenital and acquired amputations.

3   Develop an assessment program for a child with a unilateral amputation.

4   Develop a treatment program for a child with a unilateral amputation.

5   Discuss the role of the family in working with children with amputations.

case studies

Michael Donnagin, a 6-month-old boy, is brought to the clinic by his mother. Michael was born with a half humerus on the right side and the medial 2 toes on the right foot. He is an only child. His father is a loan officer in a bank and his mother is on leave from her job as a legal secretary.

Jenny Smith, a 6-year-old girl, has a left transfemoral femoral amputation secondary to a farm accident. The amputation was performed 4 weeks ago and followed a failed attempt to reattach the limb. She is referred to the amputee clinic for evaluation and treatment. Jenny lives with her parents and four older siblings on a medium size farm.

Mario Jonas, a 3-year-old boy, has a left longitudinal deficiency femur, partial proximal focal femoral deficiency (**PFFD**), Category D, and is referred to the amputee clinic for prosthetic fitting. He lives in a small town in Mexico with his mother and five older siblings. He has been walking on crutches. He has been referred to your clinic in the United States through an international aid organization. He has never been treated for his disability.

CASE STUDY ACTIVITIES

1 Classify Michael's amputations using appropriate terminology.
2 Compare and contrast acquired and congenital amputations.
3 Develop a preclinic evaluation plan for each child.
  a What critical data are needed to plan appropriate prosthetic rehabilitation?
  b What might the parents' concerns be at this time?
  c What information would you like to have from the parents?
4 Would you fit each of these children?
  a If yes, briefly describe the components you would use.
  b If no, justify your decision and determine your alternate plan of action.
5 Compare and contrast the prosthetic rehabilitation program for each of these children with that of an adult with a similar disability.

The habilitation of children with single or multiple limb loss is a complex, long term process involving specialists from many disciplines with training in pediatric care. This chapter provides a brief overview of this topic, offering general guidelines for the therapist who may occasionally work with a child who has lost one limb. Most physical therapists (PTs) and physical therapist assistants (PTAs), knowledgeable in the prosthetic care of adults, can provide effective therapy to a child with loss of one limb. The care of the child with multiple limb deficiencies requires considerable expertise and such children should be referred to special centers for optimal care.

PTs and PTAs need to be cognizant that the child is not a miniature adult. Children have special problems of developmental tasks and of parental adjustment, as well as their own adjustment and acceptance. The rehabilitation program involves the whole family, and the attitude of the parents, other siblings, and family members has considerable influence on the adjustment of the child. Children who are born without a limb or part of a limb usually adjust to limb replacement on the basis of comfort and utility. Their major goal is to emulate their peers and to participate in the activities of other children. Children who are born without one or more limbs are very adaptable; if their hands are missing, they will learn to use their feet. Prosthetic replacements must fit a functional need to be used.[1]

Children with acquired amputations, unless very young, have a sense of loss. Their acceptance of a prosthesis is usually also influenced by function and by the attitude of parents and siblings. In general, children with lower limb amputations adjust to a prosthesis better than those with upper limb loss. The higher the level of upper limb loss, the more complicated the prosthesis and the more difficult the adjustment.[1] Function and cosmesis are important considerations in acceptance of upper limb prostheses; they are basically tools and must provide greater function than the residual limb to be acceptable.[2,3]

Classification

Juvenile amputations are classified into two broad categories, acquired and congenital. Acquired amputations occur after birth and result from trauma, tumor, infection, or disease. There are approximately twice as many acquired amputations from trauma as from disease, and more acquired than congenital am-

T A B L E 1 1 . 1 **LONGITUDINAL CONGENITAL LIMB DEFICIENCIES**

Limb Segment	Bone Segment (UE) May Be Partial or Complete	Bone Segment (LE) May Be Partial or Complete
Proximal	Humeral (Hu)	Femoral (Fe)
Distal	Radial (Ra)	Tibial (Ti)
Distal	Central (Ce)	Central (Ce)
	Carpal (Ca): if partial, indicate row left.	Tarsal (Ta): if partial, indicate row left.
	Metacarpal (MC): if partial, indicate ray left.	Metatarsal (MT): if partial, indicate ray left.
	Phalangeal (Ph): if partial, indicate phalanx left.	Phalangeal (Ph): if partial, indicate phalanx left.
Combined	Indicate bone segments that remain.	Indicate bone segments which remain.
	Indicate if partial or complete.	Indicate if partial or complete.
	Indicate specific carpal, ray, or phalanx left.	Indicate specific carpal, ray, or phalanx left.

putations, although exact current figures are not available. Most traumatic amputations are the result of accidents with power tools, lawnmowers, or farm implements. The major disease causing amputations is cancer, although this number is dwindling as limb sparing surgery has become more common.[4]

Congenital amputations result from prenatal or birth defects. Many congenital amputations require subsequent surgical amputation for conversion of the anomaly to enable better prosthetic fitting. A different nomenclature is used for congenital amputations than for acquired juvenile amputations. The International Standards Organization (ISO) has developed a classification scheme for limb deficiencies present at birth based on skeletal elements (Table 11.1).

Limb deficiencies are classified as transverse or longitudinal. Transverse deficiencies are described by the level at which the limb terminates. The limb is normal proximally to the level named; distally, there is no skeletal component. A child lacking all skeletal components below the elbow has a transverse total forearm loss. If part of the bone is present, as when all components below the middle of the femur are lost, it is classified as transverse middle femoral loss.

Longitudinal deficiencies refer to those with a reduction or absence of skeletal components with normal components present below the affected part. Identification of longitudinal anomalies includes (1) the name of the affected bones in a proximal to distal order; (2) indication of whether each bone is partially or totally absent; (3) an indication of the amount of absent bone; and (4) mention of those digits, metacarpals, metatarsals, or phalanges that are present. For example, an individual with a normal tibia attached directly to the pelvis, no fibula, and the first two rays of the foot is described as having longitudinal femoral fibular deficiency with two partial rays.[5]

Congenital anomalies vary. A vestigial component may be attached to a proximal part, digits may not be separated, and individuals may sustain multiple limb deficiencies or anomalies. An innovative and creative approach to surgical interventions and fitting is used by members of child limb deficient clinics.

PROXIMAL FEMORAL FOCAL DEFICIENCIES

One special problem that is seen with some regularity is the longitudinal deficiency femur with partial PFFD. PFFD is classified in relation to the position of the foot, the condition of the hip joint, and the length of the femoral and tibial segments. This deficiency of the proximal end of the femur is characterized by a very short femoral segment that is held in flexion, abduction, and external rotation. The quadriceps muscle is frequently hypoplastic with a correspondingly small or vestigial patella. Associated ipsilateral paraxial fibular hemimelia is often present. The total limb length of the affected side is at about the same level as the knee joint on the unaffected side. The condition may be bilateral or unilateral. Variations of PFFD can be differentiated radiographically after the child is 9 to 12 months old.[6]

Representative anomalies are discussed briefly later in this chapter.

Surgical Interventions

The aim of amputation surgery, if performed, is to produce a limb that is adequate for a prosthesis and that will remain adequate through the remaining growth period and adulthood. Lower limb surgery should allow pain free weight bearing, stability, an adequately sensate limb, near normal gait, maximum bone growth, and satisfactory cosmesis. Amputation for cosmetic reasons alone should not be done until the child is old enough to share in the decision.

The child who has a traumatic or surgically elected amputation should be placed on a carefully planned postoperative program that includes exercises and activities to prevent contractures and to maintain the function of the residual limb. Parents should be informed of the effect contractures have on the usefulness of the prosthesis. Parents also need instruction in a home program, which may include assisting the child to use the anomalous limb to perform functional activities in an atypical manner.

UPPER EXTREMITY

Reconstructive surgery is frequently used to improve congenital deformities. Function and, to a lesser extent, cosmesis are the primary concerns. The surgeon must consider bone loss and incompletely developed muscles and ligaments that may affect joint function. In the upper extremity, reconstructive surgery plays a major role in the management of **syndactyly** and **polydactyly,** as well as radial and ulnar deficiencies that lead to poorly positioned hands. Surgery should be performed early and is designed to provide the child with as functional a hand as possible. Amputation of a functionless part is performed if it will enhance function. Procedures are designed to improve both function and appearance, rather than to enhance prosthetic fitting. Prostheses are designed to adapt to the limb.[7]

LOWER EXTREMITY

In the lower extremity, reconstructive surgery is often delayed to allow the greatest possible amount of bone growth. Maintenance of long bone growth plates allows the greatest development of limb length.[8] Individuals with short proximal skeletal pieces may eventually develop a usable residual limb. Severe deformities that interfere with early fitting or with function require early surgical intervention. The surgeon considers overall function and related muscular development. Progressive deformities that may occur as a result of muscle and nerve imbalances must be prevented.

Hemimelias

Hemimelias are longitudinal deficiencies in which all or part of one long bone is missing. In the lower extremity, tibial, fibular, or femoral hemimelias are possible. Fibular hemimelia results in leg length discrepancy and bowing of the tibia. Surgical lengthening of the leg has met with minimal success. Surgical arrest of the growth plate of the other limb has also been used. More recently, the Ilizarov technique[9] has met with some success. This technique involves progressive fracturing of the tibia with callus distraction and limb protection. The limb is maintained in a rigid external apparatus during this sometimes protracted process. The child is fitted with a shoe lift to equalize leg length until he or she is old enough for the lengthening procedure. Leg lengthening cannot be used if the expected discrepancy is likely to be more than 7.5 centimeters. In such cases, Syme's amputation is usually performed.[8] If the foot is removed at an early age because of unfittable deformity, then Syme's amputation will become a transtibial amputation as the child grows (Fig. 11.1).

Tibial hemimelias are usually treated with knee disarticulation amputation.[8] If part of the tibia remains, it is sometimes possible to attach the fibula to the remnant of the tibia, then perform an ankle disarticulation.

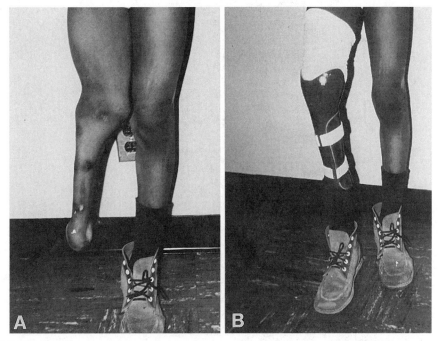

FIGURE 11.1
(*A*) Syme's amputation in infancy will become a transtibial level amputation as the child grows. (*B*) A Syme type prosthesis is still needed because of the larger distal end.

Amelias

Amelia, the total absence of a limb, may be unilateral or bilateral. Amelias are usually treated like a disarticulation. Remaining digits may be kept if they can be useful to provide sensory input or perform self care activities.

Treatment of Proximal Femoral Focal Deficiency

Treatment of PFFD is long term and may involve surgical reconstruction as well as prosthetic fitting. As the child grows, the length of the affected limb becomes progressively shorter. One method of management involves fitting the limb with an adapted prosthesis until maximal bone growth has occurred and reconstructive surgery can be performed (Fig. 11.2). After the child has reached the teen years, the knee may be fused and a Syme's amputation may be performed to provide a functional transfemoral residual limb. On some occasions, a Van Ness 180 degree rotational osteotomy of the tibia is performed that allows the ankle to be used as a knee joint and the child to be fitted with a transtibial prosthesis.[10,11] In cases of bilateral PFFD associated with upper extremity deficiencies, the feet may not be removed because the child may learn to use the feet for prehension.[8] Some clinics advocate early ablation of the foot.

This discussion may lead the reader to believe that most congenital anomalies are single bone problems, but this is rarely the case. There may be asso-

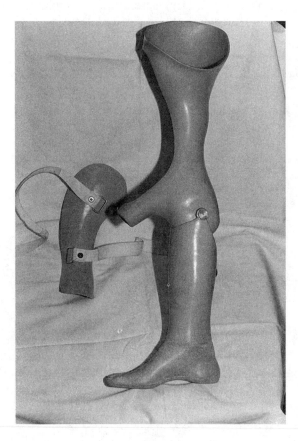

FIGURE 11.2
Prosthesis for proximal focal femoral deficiency.

ciated deformities of the lower segments of the involved limb, involvement of other extremities, and related loss of muscles and ligaments. Surgical intervention is individualized; prosthetic fitting is adapted to the residuum and the total needs of the child. Surgery may be performed early or late depending on the state of bone growth and the potential for a functional outcome.

ACQUIRED AMPUTATIONS

The surgical procedures used in acquired amputations are much like those seen in adults. Special considerations in relation to amputation surgery in children relate to bone growth.

Terminal Overgrowth

Bone overgrowth occurs most often in the femur, fibula, tibia, and humerus, especially if the amputation is through the growth areas. This is one reason why disarticulation amputations are recommended. Radiologically, the overgrowth appears as a sharp spicule of poorly trabeculated bone that extends from the end of the cut bone. Irritation of the soft tissue sometimes produces a bursa. Bone overgrowth occurs more often following acquired amputations or amputations to convert anomalies. Multiple surgical revisions may be required before bone maturity if overgrowth does occur and capping is unsuccessful. Full thickness skin coverage is desirable at the end of growing bones for comfortable prosthetic fit. This problem occurs in 8% to 12% of cases.[4,8]

Bone Spurs

Bone spurs are small bony spicules that may develop at the edge of the bone end. Spurs rarely cause problems in children and must be differentiated from overgrowth.

Adventitious Bursa

Adventitious bursa may develop in the soft tissue over an area of terminal overgrowth. It may be treated by steroid injection, socket modification, or aspiration, but permanent relief usually necessitates surgical excision of the bursa and underlying bone.

Scarring

Frequent surgical reconstructive surgery may lead to scarring of the residual limb. This rarely causes problems in the prosthetic fitting of children.

Prosthetic Fitting

The prosthesis for a congenital amputation is generally fitted as early as possible, consistent with motor development, to enable the child to meet the motor milestones. An upper extremity prosthesis is indicated when the child begins bilateral activities (between 3 and 5 months) and a lower extremity prosthesis is indicated when the child demonstrates the desire to stand (usually when the child is between 6 and 9 months). For an acquired amputation, the prosthesis is fitted as soon as the residual limb heals. The early prosthesis may be a simple bracelike device. The goal should be to provide a prosthesis that is functional and acceptable to touch and sight.

UPPER EXTREMITY

Many children with a congenital upper extremity amputation are fitted with a soft and well padded passive mitten to avoid injury to themselves and others. The early prosthesis is not powered and is suspended by a simple chest harness. As the child develops motor control, a padded hook may substitute for the mitten and eventually be attached to a cable for power. Early prostheses need to be simple, but as children grow, they need to try different terminal devices to determine what is most functional. Myoelectric prostheses become an option for children 18 months and older; the myoelectric hand has voluntary control of both opening and closing and possesses stronger pinch force than the cable-controlled hook. It operates independently of elbow position. However, it is heavier, it cannot be placed in water, and the cosmetic glove requires regular replacement. Young children adapt to myoelectric prostheses fairly readily depending on their motor development. The child's size and degree of development also affect the selection of components, because not all components are made in all sizes.

Children with unilateral upper extremity loss become dominant on the unamputated side. Some become adept at using the residual limb for bilateral activities and may reject the prosthesis. Early fitting for both congenital and acquired amputations helps the child integrate the prosthesis into daily life.

It is important to consider appearance as well as function when selecting components for children with upper extremity loss. Children need to fit in with their peers in both activity and looks; the more cosmetic the prosthesis, the better are its chances of acceptance. Children grow fast and prostheses require new parts, sockets, and components on a regular basis. Using multilayered sockets and heavy socks expands the life of prosthetic sockets.[12] Finally, components need to be durable to support an active lifestyle. Upper extremity prosthetic components are discussed in greater detail in Chapter 10.

LOWER EXTREMITY

Lower extremity prostheses must also support developmental activities. As in the upper extremity, simplicity and durability are important in selecting components. Cosmesis becomes important in the teen years for both boys and girls. Generally, the child with a unilateral lower extremity amputation is fitted when ready to pull to stand. There is little point in fitting earlier because rolling and crawling can usually be done more easily without a prosthesis and suspension is very difficult to attain. The major considerations in fitting an infant are to select a socket that will allow for linear and circumferential growth and to provide suspension without interfering with the child's activity. Complex prosthetic feet and prosthetic knee joints are not necessary for children who are just beginning to walk. Some very young children with transtibial amputations may slip out of a patellar-tendon-bearing (PTB) prosthesis and require a corset for suspension. The infant with a transfemoral amputation is fitted without a knee joint. The child with a hip disarticulation is fitted with a hip joint to allow sitting, but no knee joint. When the child begins to gain control, a manual lock knee may be used as a transition to a fully articulated limb. Feet in children's sizes are available for 6-month-old infants. Knee units are manufactured for 2-year-old children. Hydraulic knee mechanisms and suction sockets are usually not used until the child is 10 years or older.

Children with limb anomalies and partial limb remnants require adaptation of standard sockets. Radiographs are taken before prosthetic fitting to determine the bony structure of the incomplete extremity. Subsequent radiographs allow assessment of development for required prosthetic modifications as the child grows. The child must be followed closely to avoid skin problems and socket discomfort resulting from growth. Bone growth in the congenitally deficient limb will likely be diminished, at least in part, because of abnormal, asymmetric, or reduced muscle pull and weight bearing. Children with PFFD are fitted with adapted ischial weight-bearing prostheses. If the foot remains, it is placed in plantar flexion to fit more cosmetically, while allowing some weight bearing on the bottom of the foot.[13] Alignment techniques for the child's prosthesis are similar to those for the adult's prosthesis.

In cases of bilateral involvement, when both limbs terminate at or above the knee, stubbies (see Chaps. 5 and 7) may be used in the transitional stage. Stubbies consist of sockets with foot pieces that usually have a rocker bottom that is slightly elongated posteriorly. A Silesian bandage is usually sufficient for suspension unless the residual limbs are short, in which case a pelvic band with hip joints is used. Shoulder straps may be used in children under 5 years of age because bilateral pelvic bands limit hip motion. The socket is flexed a few degrees to prevent excessive lumbar lordosis. Stubbies are indicated as an initial prescription when the child is too young for secure balance or longer articulated prostheses as a primary fitting.

MULTIPLE LIMB LOSS

Children with multiple limb loss or limb anomalies require adapted sockets and components and are usually treated through juvenile amputee programs. The number of children born with congenital limb deficiencies increased exponentially in the 1950s and 1960s as a result of the effects of Thalidomide.[14,15] New surgical techniques and new prosthetic and mobility aids were developed to help these children achieve as much function as possible. Special juvenile amputee clinics throughout the country are important resources, especially for children with multiple congenital deformities.[16]

SPORTS PROSTHESES

Sports and other vigorous activities are an important part of a child's development. Prostheses need to be durable enough to withstand the stress of strenuous activities as well as protect both the child and any opponents from injury. Many recreational programs are available for children with limb deficiencies. Various adaptations can be constructed to aid in sports activities. Adapted skis are common for children and adults. Old prostheses can be made usable in water for fishing or rafting. Special rotators allow translatory movements in both upper and lower extremities.[17] Many sports activities require no special prosthesis. PTs and PTAs who may work with children need to be aware of the potential for participation in sports.

Training

Working with children with limb loss really means working with parents. The parents have the prime responsibility for helping the child adjust to the prosthesis, learn to incorporate it into daily life, and accept himself or herself as a person who has a limb loss. As the child grows, peer acceptance becomes important. Children with congenital or acquired amputations may be at risk for long term psychological and social maladjustment. The long term stress of coping with a handicap that limits function sets the person apart and makes daily life difficult. Varni et al.[18] studied a group of children with congenital and acquired limb loss and suggested that children with low levels of support from peers, family, and teachers were at greater risk for symptoms of depression and low self esteem. Early referral of parents and children for evaluation and social services is recommended. Some prosthetists and therapists have used amputee dolls to help children understand prosthetic replacements. Svoboda[19] created a series of dolls with various limbs missing as well as miniature prostheses. Children are encouraged to play with these dolls to act out their feelings and gain a better understanding of prosthetic replacements.

Upper extremity prosthetic training is usually performed by occupational therapists. Children learn fairly easily as long as the training is at a level appropriate to their development and the activities are interesting. Most children require minimal training in the use of lower extremity prosthetic devices. The parents should be given systematic instruction in the therapy program with regular review since they will continue with it at home. Play is the primary motivation for desired movements and activity. Therapists must be careful not to expect more from the child than from peers with normal extremity function. The normal child does not establish heel to toe gait until about 2 years of age. At about 20 months, the normal child can stand on one foot with help, at 3 years on one foot momentarily, at 4 years for several seconds, and at 5 years for longer periods.

The knee of the transfemoral prosthesis is nonarticulated or locked until the child is secure in stiff legged walking. Prosthetic heel strike to toe off gait is not usually attained until the child is about 5 years old or can demonstrate sustained one legged standing. Efforts to develop a smooth alternating progression should follow. The major causes of gait deviations are growth or worn prosthetic parts.

Children grow longitudinally and circumferentially. A new prosthesis is indicated when the old prosthesis is more than 1 centimeter (about $\frac{3}{8}$ inch) too short. A delay in the replacement of a short prosthesis may result in the development of scoliosis. A new prosthesis or socket is required about every 1 to 2 years for circumferential growth. Follow up is usually necessary every 3 to 6 months but may need to be more frequent during adolescent growth spurts. Parents must be instructed in, and responsible for, the care of the residual limb and prosthesis for the young child.

CASE STUDIES

Michael Donnagin: Michael's evaluation involves mostly play as you determine his developmental level. He may already be using the residual limb for bilateral activities. A great deal of information regarding his parents' attitude toward the disability and the potential support for therapeutic activities can be gathered through an informal interview. Michael would be expected to develop normally and should be ready for initial fitting with a nonarticulated arm with a soft passive hand. The loss of toes will not limit his standing and walking when he is ready and may not be a problem throughout his life. It will probably be helpful to the parents to talk to other parents with children in the clinic. Because they may have a tendency to be overprotective, it would be helpful to remind them early that Michael is a boy first and a handicapped child second.

Jenny Smith: Jenny's evaluation will be similar to that of an adult with a transfemoral amputation. You will need information on the residual limb and hip range of motion and strength. It will be important to determine when the limb will be ready for fitting because it is desirable to fit a child as soon as possible. Residual limb wrapping may not be an issue unless there is considerable edema. Jenny probably learned to walk on crutches while still in the hospital. The attitudes of both the parents and the child are critical, particularly if the parents blame themselves for the accident. Trauma is associated with the failed replantation. Jenny and her parents may have many questions that will need to be answered fully. When the residual limb is fully healed and free of edema, Jenny can be fitted with a lightweight transfemoral prosthesis, probably with a constant friction knee and SACH foot. She will need some gait training and would be expected to do well with the prosthesis.

Mario Jonas: Mario's needs for prosthetic care and replacement are dictated to some degree by where he lives and how often he will be able to return to the clinic. Depending on the extent of leg length differences and whether the foot is usable, he may be fitted with an adapted PFFD prosthesis with the foot encased and used for partial weight bearing. It is too early to consider amputation of the foot. The family will need to learn how to care for the prosthesis and what to do as the child grows. Again, the parents are the pivotal partners in the care of the child and need to be kept as fully informed as possible.

SUMMARY

Care of the child with an amputation is a specialized type of practice that usually can be best carried out by a pediatric amputee clinic team, particularly when working with a child with multiple limb deficiencies. Many resources exist for the PT or PTA who only occasionally encounters a child, such as the Association of Children's Prosthetic-Orthotic Clinics. The child's developmental needs must be considered if prosthetic replacements and management are to be used to enhance the child's normal development as much as possible. Many children use nonstandard prostheses. Creativity is needed in defining one or more functional limbs. The parents are integral members of the rehabilitation team and need to be involved in all aspects of care.

GLOSSARY

Adventitious bursa	A fluid-filled sac, usually around a joint, that develops in response to friction or pressure.
Amelia	Congenital absence of one or more limbs.
Anomalous	A deviation from normal.
Hemimelia	Longitudinal deficiencies in which all or part of one long bone is missing.
Hypoplastic	Defective development of tissues.
Myoelectric	Muscle movement that is stimulated by electricity.
PFFD	Proximal focal femoral deficiency.
Polydactyly	Multiple congenital abnormalities of the hand and wrist.
Spicule	A thin sliver of bone.
Syndactyly	The congenital joining of digits.
Vestigial	A small, incompletely developed structure.

REFERENCES

1. Fisk, JR: Introduction to the child amputee. In Bowker, JH, and Michael, JW (eds.): Atlas of Limb Prosthetics: Surgical, Prosthetic, and Rehabilitation Principles, ed. 2. Mosby-Year Book, St. Louis, 1992, pp. 731–734.
2. Patterson, DB: Acceptance rate of myoelectric prosthesis. J Assoc Child Prosthet Orthot Clin 25:73–76, 1990.
3. Weaver, SA: Comparison of myoelectric and conventional prostheses for adolescent amputees. Am J Occup Ther 42:78–91, 1988.
4. Tooms, RE: Acquired amputation in children. In Bowker, JH, and Michael, JW (eds.): Atlas of Limb Prosthetics: Surgical, Prosthetic, and Rehabilitation Principles, ed. 2. Mosby-Year Book, St. Louis, 1992, pp. 735–742.
5. Day, HJB: The ISO/ISPO classification of congenital limb deficiency. In Bowker, JH, and Michael, JW (eds.): Atlas of Limb Prosthetics: Surgical, Prosthetic and Rehabilitation Principles, ed. 2. Mosby-Year Book, St. Louis, 1992, pp. 743–748.
6. Aitken, GT: Proximal femoral focal deficiency: Definition, classification, and management. In Proximal Femoral Focal Deficiency: A Congenital Anomaly, NAS 1734. National Academy of Sciences, Washington, DC, 1969.
7. Light, T: Upper-limb deficiencies: surgical management. In Bowker, JH, and Michael, JW (eds.): Atlas of Limb Prosthetics: Surgical, Prosthetic, and Rehabilitation Principles, ed. 2. Mosby-Year Book, St. Louis, 1992, pp. 749–760.
8. Kruger, LM: Lower-limb deficiencies: Surgical management. In Bowker, JH, and Michael, JW (eds.): Atlas of Limb Prosthetics: Surgical, Prosthetic, and Rehabilitation Principles, ed. 2. Mosby-Year Book, St. Louis, 1992, pp. 795–834.
9. Frankel, VH, and Lloyd-Roberts, GC: The Ilizarov technique. Bull Hosp Jt Dis Orthop Inst 48:17–27, 1988.
10. Cummings, DR, and Kapp, SL: Lower-limb pediatric prosthetics: General considerations and philosophy. J Pediatr Orthop 4:196–206, 1992.
11. Aitken, GT: The child with an acquired amputation. InterClinic Information Bulletin 7:1–15, 1968.
12. Supan, T: Upper limb deficiencies: Prosthetic and orthotic management. In Bowker, JH, and Michael, JW (eds.): Atlas of Limb Prosthetics: Surgical, Prosthetic, and Rehabilitation Principles, ed. 2. Mosby-Year Book, St. Louis, 1992, pp. 761–766.
13. Oglesby, DG, Jr, and Tablada, C: Lower limb deficiencies: Prosthetic and orthotic management. In Bowker, JH, and Michael, JW (eds.): Atlas of Limb Prosthetics: Surgical, Prosthetic, and Rehabilitation Principles, ed. 2. Mosby-Year Book, St. Louis, 1992, pp. 835–838.

14. Marquardt, E: The management of infants with malformation of the extremities. In Limb Development and Deformity: Problems of Evaluation and Rehabilitation. Charles C Thomas, Springfield, IL, 1969.
15. McBride, WG: Thalidomide and congenital abnormalities. Lancet 2:1358, 1961.
16. Marquardt, E: The multiple-limb-deficient child. In Bowker, JH, and Michael, JW (eds.): Atlas of Limb Prosthetics: Surgical, Prosthetic, and Rehabilitation Principles. Mosby-Year Book, St. Louis, 1992.
17. Page, CJ, and Messner, DG: Juvenile amputees: Sports and recreation program development. In Bowker, JH, and Michael, JW (eds.): Atlas of Limb Prosthetics: Surgical, Prosthetic, and Rehabilitation Principles. Mosby-Year Book, St. Louis, 1992.
18. Varni, JW, Setoguchi, Y, Rappaport, R, and Talbot, D: Effects of stress, social support and self esteem on depression in children with limb deficiencies. Arch Phys Med Rehabil 72:1053–1058, 1991.
19. Svoboda, J: Psychosocial considerations in pediatrics: Use of amputee dolls. Journal of Prosthetics and Orthotics 4:207–212, 1992.

Index

The letter f following a page number indicates a figure; the letter t indicates a table.

Movement transition(s), 91
MRI. *See* Magnetic resonance imaging (MRI)
Multiaxis knee joint(s), 132, 136
Multiflex ankle system, 133
Multilayered socket(s), 226
Multilevel tourniquet test, 25
Multiple limb deficiencies, children and, 220–221, 227, 229
Muscle(s), 8, 38, 41, 86
    ankle foot mechanisms and, 112–113
    children and, 222–223, 225, 227
    exercises and, 89–90
    lower limb amputation and, 54, 57–59, 63–64
    postoperative evaluation of, 72–73
    terminal devices and, 209, 214
    weakness in, 11, 79
Musculoskeletal examination, diabetic foot and, 41
Myodesis, 5, 8
    definition, 13, 65
    lower limb amputation and, 54, 58–59
Myoelectric, definition, 137, 217, 230
Myoelectric control(s), 11, 136, 217
    upper limb prostheses with, 206, 208t, 209–211, 211t, 212, 214
    children and, 226, 230
    transradial, 209f, 213, 215f
    wrist units, 216–217
Myoplasty
    definition, 13, 65
    lower limb amputation and, 54, 58–59

Narrow based gait, 157–158
National Wheelchair and Amputee Championships, 198f
Necrosis, 21, 144.
    definition, 50
    diabetic foot and, 39, 43, 45
Neuroarthropathy, 41
    definition, 50
Neurological examination, diabetic foot and, 40–41
Neuroma(s), 75
    definition, 65
    lower limb amputation and, 53, 68, 145
Neuropathic ulcer(s), 45
Neuropathy, 34, 37–38, 50
    definition, 34, 50
Nonarticulated arm, 229
Nondynamic response prosthetic feet, 113–114

Occupational therapist(s), 228
One legged standing, 173, 228
Onychogryphosis, 45
Open environment(s), 181–182, 184f
Orthotic device(s), diabetic foot and, 44, 49

Orthotic rehabilitation, 9–10
Osteomyelitis, lower limb amputation and, 58–59
Osteophyte formation, 58

Outcome(s), 143, 172, 183
Outdoor activities, 197. *See also* Recreational activities; Sports
Outrigger(s), 197
Outset foot, 155–157

Padded hook, 226
Pain, 26, 40, 89, 94, 145. *See also* Phantom pain
    postoperative dressings and, 68–69, 72
        upper limb amputations and, 204–205, 217
    lower extremity prostheses and, 150, 153, 160, 165
    residual limb and, 94
Palmar flexion, 211–212
Paré, Ambroise, 4, 6
    above-knee artificial leg invented by, 5f
Parental reaction to congenital anomaly, 103, 220, 228–229
Parmelee, Dubois D., 7
    suction socket prosthesis of, 7f
Parallel bars, 183
Paraolympics, 198, 199f
Partial foot amputation(s), 112, 115–117
Partial limb remnant(s), 227
Passive hand(s), 207–208, 208t, 209, 211t
    children and, 229
Passive mitten, 226
Patella, 63, 96
Patellar tendon bearing (PTB) prosthesis, 3f, 9, 118, 150, 226
    liner in, 118f, 119–120
    pressure and relief areas for, 119t
    suspension mechanisms for, 120t
Patellar tendon supracondylar suprapatellar (PTSCSP) prostheses, 153
Patency, lower extremity amputation and, 53, 56
    definition, 65
Pelvic band, 129, 130f, 166, 169, 227
Pelvic displacement, 154
Peripheral sympathetic neuropathy, 37
Peripheral vascular disease(s), 10, 15–34
    case studies, 16, 27–30
    client education programs, 31t, 94
    etiology, pathology, and major symptoms of, 20t
    intermittent pressure application to leg, 33f
    lower extremity amputation and, 53, 55
Personality, effect on adjustment to amputation, 100, 102